HOSPITAL HISTORY AND MEDICAL PRACTICE IN MY SMALL TOWN

with

Personal Stories of the Author

By

Albert H. Meinke, Jr., M.D.

Trafford Publishing Company

National Library of Canada Cataloguing in Publication Data

Meinke, Albert H., 1919-
Hospital history and medical practice in my small town : with personal stories of the author / Albert H. Meinke, Jr.
ISBN 1-55395-745-8
1. Meinke, Albert H., 1919- 2. Physicians--Michigan--Eaton Rapids--Biography. I. Title.
R250.E28M44 2003 610'.92 C2003-900542-9

TRAFFORD

This book was published *on-demand* in cooperation with Trafford Publishing.
On-demand publishing is a unique process and service of making a book available for retail sale to the public taking advantage of on-demand manufacturing and Internet marketing. **On-demand publishing** includes promotions, retail sales, manufacturing, order fulfilment, accounting and collecting royalties on behalf of the author.

Suite 6E, 2333 Government St., Victoria, B.C. V8T 4P4, CANADA
Phone 250-383-6864 Toll-free 1-888-232-4444 (Canada & US)
Fax 250-383-6804 E-mail sales@trafford.com
Web site www.trafford.com TRAFFORD PUBLISHING IS A DIVISION OF TRAFFORD HOLDINGS LTD.
Trafford Catalogue #03-0108 www.trafford.com/robots/03-0108.html

10 9 8 7 6 5 4

ABOUT THE AUTHOR

Dr. Albert H. Meinke, Jr. was born on September 26, 1919 in Detroit, Michigan, where he attended the public schools, and graduated in 1937 with honors from Thomas M. Cooley High School. He then attended Albion College in Albion, Michigan, where he earned a Bachelor of Arts Degree in June 1941. He received his Doctor of Medicine Degree from the University of Michigan Medical School in October 1943. That unusual time of year for a graduation came about because the United States had formally entered World War II on December 7, 1941, and the university promptly adopted an accelerated medical curriculum with three full semesters of classes each calendar year. Immediately after graduation from medical school he began a nine-month rotating internship at Edward W. Sparrow Hospital in Lansing, Michigan. A few days before the internship was finished, on July 29, 1944, he married Edmere L. Bondesen of Detroit. The next few days were spent in Lansing finishing up hospital clinical records, and on August 2, 1944 he entered active duty in the Army of the United States as a First Lieutenant in the Medical Corps.

After going through an extensive training course for new medical officers at the Army Medical Field Service School at Carlisle Barracks, Pennsylvania, he was assigned to the Army School of Tropical Medicine at Moore General Hospital in Swannanoa, North Carolina, where he studied tropical diseases, and also served as a ward officer in the hospital. His patients were soldiers suffering with tropical diseases contracted in the South Pacific, and this led him to believe that he would be treating such tropical diseases later on in his tour of duty.

After this initial training was finished, he was surprised to find that the Army, in its great wisdom, assigned him as a Battalion Surgeon in the U.S. Tenth Mountain Division, --- the only division of ski troops in the entire U. S. armed forces. In this capacity he served front line infantrymen through the Division's entire combat period in Italy, and remained in the Division until it was deactivated in the late fall of 1945.

In late August of 1946, Dr. Meinke moved to Eaton Rapids, Michigan to take over the medical practice of another physician who had been a missionary doctor in Africa and had been recalled during the War to serve Eaton Rapids, because at that time all of the town's able-bodied, practicing physicians were away, serving in the armed forces.

In 1984, at the age of sixty-five, Dr. Meinke retired, and moved with his wife to Kewadin, Michigan into a home on the shore of Torch Lake. There he wrote the book MOUNTAIN TROOPS AND MEDICS, which tells the story of his wartime experiences in the Ski Troops. The book was well received, and is now in its second printing.

AUTHOR'S PREFACE

The idea to write about some of my practice experiences, and at the same time point out some of the changes in medicine which were taking place during all of those years, came to me in September 2001, shortly after I received an invitation to speak at the dedication ceremonies for a recently completed, large addition to the modern Eaton Rapids Medical Center. Because I had been deeply involved with its founding and early operations, and had treated patients there during the first 26 years of its existence, I was asked to speak for five to seven minutes about the early years of the hospital, ------ years when it was known as **Eaton Rapids Community Hospital**. As I was thinking about what to say, I realized that the time allotted for my speech would not allow me to even begin to adequately present the subject. Here then, in these pages, are recorded some of the many things I would have liked to have told my audience in that speech. It is my story of the hospitals and medicine in my hometown, presented truthfully, accurately, and in some detail.

In August of 1946 I chose Eaton Rapids to be the town in which I would establish my medical practice and rear my family. Although it was my intent to stay for only two or three years, and then take a residency in general surgery somewhere in order to become a board certified surgical specialist, my wife and I became so deeply and pleasantly involved with its people and its hospital that we stayed until I retired from practice 38 years later.

For an overview of the early medical history of Eaton Rapids I am indebted to one of my earliest patients, W. Scott Munn, who researched the history of the area, and wrote about it in his book, THE ONLY EATON RAPIDS ON EARTH. Munn's book was apparently self-published. It contains no mention of a copyright, and there is no ISBN Number in the book. There is merely a statement on the backside of the title page that it had been printed by Edwards Brothers, Inc. of Ann Arbor, Michigan. No publication date is given, but the author dated his autograph in my copy of the book on 8/2/52.

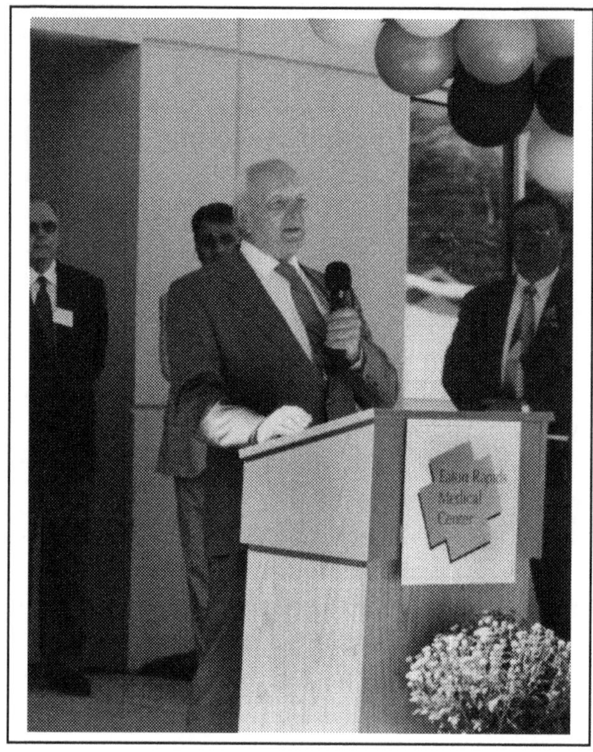

The author, Albert H. Meinke, Jr., speaking to the crowd of people on the lawn of the Eaton Rapids Medical Center on 6 September 2002, during the dedication ceremonies for the extensive new building additions.

TABLE OF CONTENTS

ABOUT THE AUTHOR v
AUTHOR'S PREFACE vii

CHAPTER I — EATON RAPIDS 13
CHAPTER II — STIMSON HOSPITAL 21
CHAPTER III — MY ARRIVAL IN TOWN 31
CHAPTER IV — MY FIRST OFFICE 35
CHAPTER V — MY PRACTICE BEGINS 39
CHAPTER VI — THE BIG SNOW AND FLOOD 55
CHAPTER VII — SWITCH TO GROUP PRACTICE 65
CHAPTER VIII — EARLY CHANGES IN MEDICAL PRACTICE 69
CHAPTER IX — STIMSON HOSPITAL CONDEMNED ... 81
CHAPTER X — THE BIRTH OF A NEW HOSPITAL 85
CHAPTER XI — THE TRANSITION 93
CHAPTER XII — EATON RAPIDS COMMUNITY HOSPITAL 97
CHAPTER XIII — REGULATOR PROBLEMS 103
CHAPTER XIV — MEDICAL INSURANCE 107
CHAPTER XV — EATON RAPIDS MEDICAL CLINIC 117
CHAPTER XVI — OBSTETRIC SERVICES 125
CHAPTER XVII — ANESTHESIA 133
CHAPTER XVIII — EMERGENCY SERVICES 143
CHAPTER XIX — THE CORONER SYSTEM 147
CHAPTER XX — HOUSECALL ADVENTURES 155

- A Dermatology Lesson 156
- Goose Attack 157
- Redecorating Anyone? 159
- Bogged Down 159
- A Birth in "Squalor City" 161
- A Problem in Logistics 162
- The Tale of a Crazy Woman 164

CHAPTER XXI — OFFICE STORIES 169

- Dermatology to the Rescue 169
- Cookies Anyone? 171
- An Imagined Catastrophe 172
- Success Through Procrastination 173
- Tattoo Tale No. 1 175

Tattoo Tale No. 2 176
Tattoo Tale No. 3 176

CHAPTER XXII EMERGENCY ROOM STORIES 179
Sudden Anaphylaxis 179
Chinese Water Torture 180
Severe Burns 181
Lacerated Ear 182
Death of a Child 183
Endotracheal Intubation 183
The Tale of Mister Lucky 185
Those Damn Cows!!!! 189
Shell Fragments??? 191
Quick Draw? 192
Is he dead yet? 193

CHAPTER XXIII HOSPITAL INPATIENT STORIES ... 197
The Tub Bath 197
Liquid Appendectomy 197
Acute Myocardial Infarction 200
Refrigeration Anesthesia 203
A Strange Case of FUO 207
Chiropractor Referrals 209
Odors in Medical Practice 211

CHAPTER XXIV FOREIGN BODY STORIES 215
A Surgical Tool 217
Buckshot, Glass and Other Things ... 218
The Lost Penny 219
The Swallowed Chain 220
Another Case Not Appendicitis 221
Foreign Bodies in the Ears and Nose 222
A Record for a Foreign Body? 223

APPENDIX A by Edward B. McRee 225

HOSPITAL HISTORY AND MEDICAL PRACTICE IN MY SMALL TOWN

with
Personal Stories of the Author

CHAPTER I

EATON RAPIDS

Eaton Rapids is a lovely small town located on both sides of the Grand River in Eaton County, Michigan. A separate channel leaves the main river and rejoins it downstream, so that the greater part of downtown is actually surrounded by water, and can be considered to be an island. In its very early days there were Indian encampments on the riverbanks, and its citizens were mainly farmers, traders and individual small business people. Small gristmills and sawmills sprang up along the waterways to harness the waterpower. Small businesses were established in town, but most of them were wiped out in 1864 when a huge fire destroyed most of the downtown area. In 1869 a water well was driven into the ground in the downtown area, and when the water was found to have "magnetic" and "curative" powers, the era of mineral waters and mineral baths in Eaton Rapids began. During the next ten years a dozen more wells were drilled in the same general area, and a number of hotels sprang up to accommodate the many tourists who arrived daily to drink of the water and to take mineral baths. Eaton Rapids soon became known as THE SARATOGA OF THE WEST, after the famous Saratoga Springs area in New York, and, for many years, guests in the hotels and rooming houses outnumbered the regular residents of the town. This period of prosperity lasted some thirty years, until mineral spa treatment went out of fashion.

Eventually three woolen mills were established in Eaton Rapids, and the manufacture of woolen goods became its leading industry as raw wool was processed into finished products. One of them, the Horner Woolen Mill, made material for the upholstery used in Hudson Motor Cars, and supplied woolen blankets for one of the famous large ocean liners. Another, the Davidson Woolen Mill, made yarn, which was tightly wound on a core to make the "stuffing" of major league baseballs.

When I began practice, Main Street was lined on both sides with small stores and businesses. Most of them were old and well established, but some, like mine, were new ventures being started by veterans returning from WW II. People in the area were still farming, but many also had regular jobs away from home, and many of them regularly commuted to work in Lansing or Jackson. Eaton Rapids is conveniently located between these two cities in the southern half of the Lower Peninsula of Michigan, near the center of the "palm" of the "mitten." It is about 16 miles south of Lansing, where the highways, M-99 and M-50, join together, and about 24 miles north of Jackson, Michigan. When I first arrived the area population was said to be about 3,500 people in town, and fewer than that residing in the surrounding farmlands outside of the city limits. Today the residents living in the town number about 5,000, but the surrounding farmlands have been divided and subdivided, and so many houses have been built, so that estimates of the population living in the whole area now run as high as 40,000.

In August of 1946 when I arrived, there were six doctors actively established and practicing in Eaton Rapids.

Preston VanKolken, M.D. had been recalled by the U.S. Government from missionary work in Africa to practice in Eaton Rapids, because all of the area's vigorous and able-bodied physicians had been taken into the Armed Forces to serve in World War II. Now that the War was finished, he was anxious to return to Africa, to continue his missionary work. I agreed to buy his instruments and office equipment, and to take his place in town.

Bert VanArk, M.D. was a graduate of Rush Medical School in Chicago who had started his practice in Eaton Rapids before the United States entered World War II. He volunteered to serve in the Army during the War, although he was of an age that he might not have been called up had he declined to volunteer. Most people thought that his volunteering was very patriotic, but I had some doubts. During our long acquaintance I remember him several times saying,

"I'd rather be shot to death, than worked to death!"

Dr. Bert returned to Eaton Rapids from his wartime service to re-enter medical practice before I got out of the Army. His office was downtown on South Main Street

Herman VanArk, M.D. was a nephew to Dr. Bert VanArk. He had also been recently separated from the service, and had come to join with his uncle in medical practice. He had served in the Army, had seen combat in Europe, and had distinguished himself by earning the Silver Star Medal for gallantry in action. Because he too had been shot at in the front lines of battle, I have always felt that there was a sort of special relationship between us. He was a graduate of Marquette Medical School, and was a conservative, well-trained doctor of medicine.

Sydney Goff, M.D. was a graduate of Rush Medical School in Chicago, but he also had teaching credentials, and had taught high school chemistry for a time before he became a physician. In 1941 Dr. Goff bought the practice of Dr. Tom Wilensky, who was then practicing in Eaton Rapids. Dr. Goff soon moved his family to Eaton Rapids, and began to practice. However, about a year later he was taken in the military draft, and served the rest of WW II in the Army. He also had been separated from the service, and was back in his private practice, before I arrived in town. His office was located above some stores across the street about a block to the South of where I eventually established my office on Main Street.

J. W. Irwin, M.D. was an elderly doctor with an office in town, who had continued to practice during the war. His practice was very limited. After my arrival he did not admit patients to the hospital, and I had little contact with him. However, some twelve years later I suddenly became his attending physician. He died at an advanced age in Eaton Rapids Community Hospital shortly after it opened.

Don V. Hargrave, M.D. was a graduate of the University of Michigan Medical School who served in the U.S. armed forces in World War I, and started medical practice in Eaton Rapids sometime afterward. In addition to his medical practice he served as Health Officer for the city, and promoted the installation of an up to date sewage system.

Although their offices were located elsewhere, two other doctors of medicine also came to town occasionally to see patients. **Dr. Cyril Hanft, M.D.** practiced in the tiny town of Springport, and occasionally delivered babies in the Eaton Rapids hospital, and a **Dr. Kraft** practiced in Leslie, Michigan, but treated an occasional patient in the Eaton Rapids area.

Don F. Hutton, D.O. was an osteopathic physician who had an office in town, but did not admit patients to the local hospital. If he had hospital patients he sent them to Lansing General Hospital, which was an osteopathic hospital. Eaton Rapids also had two chiropractors, **Dr. Edward Grandy** and **Dr. H. V. Martin**. Dr Martin had his office downtown on Main Street, and would sometimes try to tease me, whenever we happened to meet, by offering to treat me in his office at no charge. Dr. Grandy owned and practiced in one of the old downtown hotels that had once been a tourist attraction because of the mineral baths it offered to the public.

Although it was a small town and had a rural atmosphere, Eaton Rapids was close enough to the Michigan State Capitol to make all of the amenities of the city of Lansing easily available to everyone who lived in the area. It also had a small, well-run, proprietary hospital, with which I felt quite comfortable. I did feel strongly that a hospital was necessary to my practice.

Among the doctors who preceded me in Eaton Rapids, and who are mentioned in Munn's book, are some about whom I heard during my practice years, either because there was something unusual in their stories, or there were descendents still living in the area. Among them were James B. Bradley, M.D., Francis M. Blanchard, M.D., Harry J. Prall, M.D., Thomas Wilensky, M.D., Dr. Wilson Canfield, and E. E. Overfield, M.D.

Dr, Wilensky was a graduate of the University of Western Ontario. He sold his practice in Eaton Rapids to take specialty training in proctology and rectal surgery, and had finished this training before I arrived in Eaton Rapids. Both he and Dr. Prall were then practicing in Lansing.

Stimson Hospital was well established and in continuous operation on the corner of Main and Plain Streets, in a building that looked like a large private mansion. According to Munn, it was built sometime in the 1870's by John T. Sweezy, and sold to Fred Spicer sometime in the 1880's. The Spicer family lived there until 1918, when Dr. Charles A. Stimson, Dr. Francis M. Blanchard, and Miss Harriet Chapman, a graduate nurse, bought the property, and remodeled the building to become the Harriet Chapman Hospital. They owned and operated it together, and at the height of its glory Harriet Chapman Hospital had a relatively large nursing staff, and included a respected school of nursing. The remodeling included the installation of an elevator large enough to easily accommodate a hospital bed, and tragedy struck in 1919 when Dr. Blanchard, stepped through the elevator door into the darkness, and fell down the elevator shaft to his death. When Harriet Chapman died in 1930, the name of the hospital changed, but the hospital continued to be operated by Dr Stimson alone. He put his nurse, Miss Bernice Bowman in charge of hospital operations, and when Dr. Stimson died in 1943, the property was inherited by his widow, Mrs. Isabel Stimson, and Miss Bowman together, who continued to operate it as Stimson Hospital.

This then was the stage upon which I stepped to begin my practice.

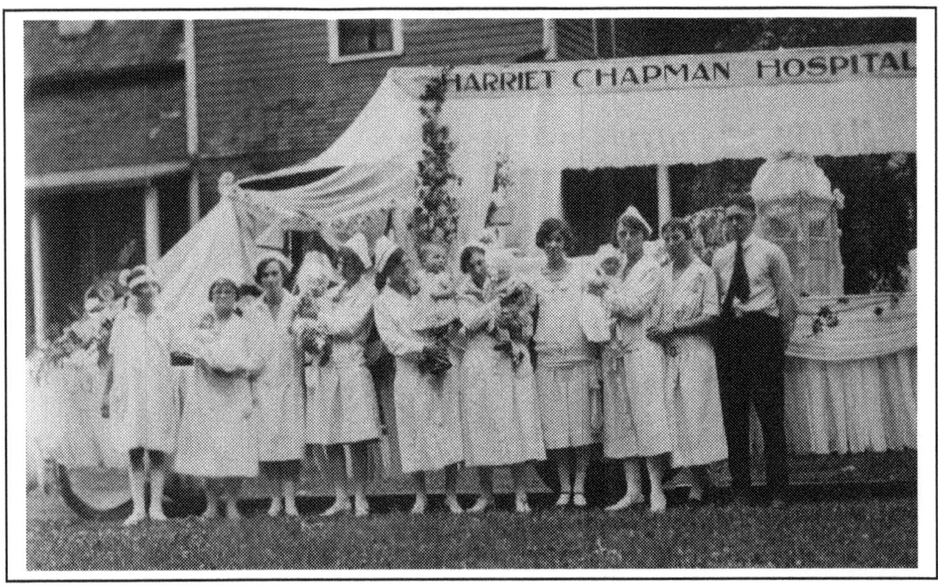

This picture, taken sometime in the mid-1920's, shows a parade float produced and sponsored by the Harriet Chapman Hospital. It probably appeared in Eaton Rapids in a parade to celebrate a national holiday such as the 4th of July. The float appears to have been built upon a farm truck or tractor, and was probably driven by the only man seen in the picture. Presumably, the nurses and nursing students rode on the float holding the babies. All of the people shown remain unidentified, but the person standing next to the driver may be Bernice Bowman, and second to the left from her may be her friend, Ruth Rider. Those women in the picture who are not wearing nurses' caps are probably students, because in those days such caps could not be worn until after graduation.

Judging from the siding and the porch post in the picture the house in the background is probably the house where the student nurses lived, and perhaps attended some classes.

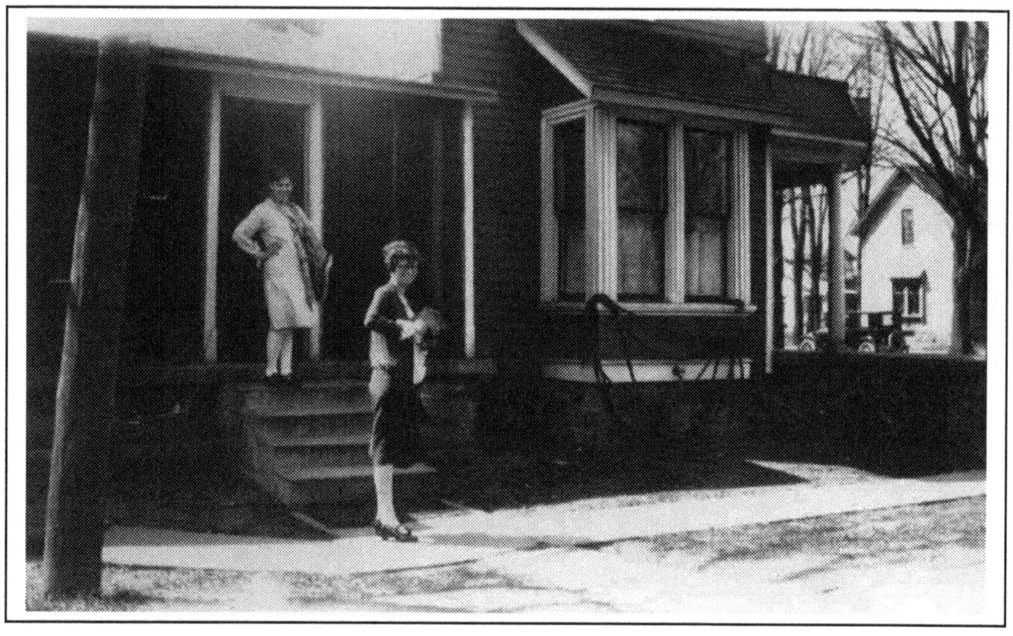

The other side of the Student Nurses' Home. Standing at the door is Bernice Bowman at the age of nineteen. Below on the sidewalk is her friend, Ruth Rider. The picture was taken in 1926.

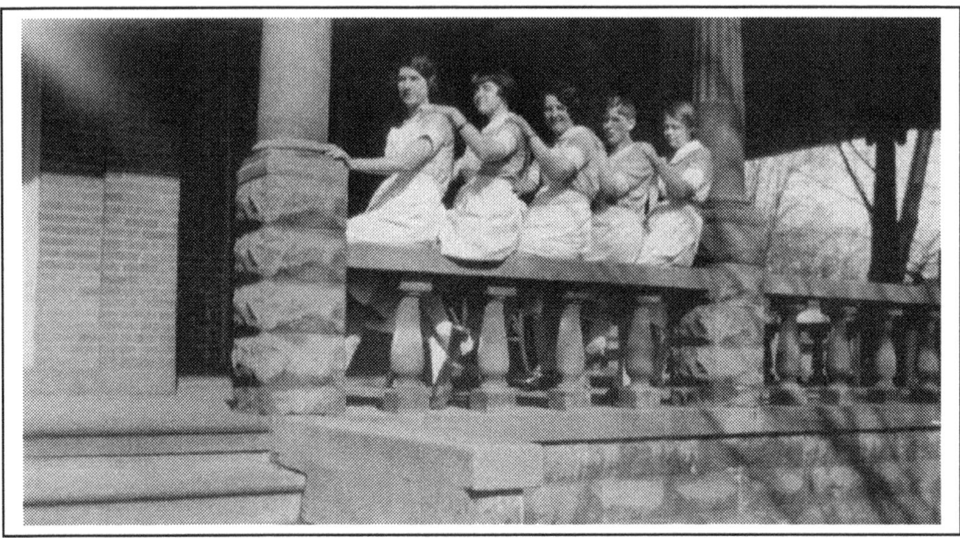

A graduating class of new nurses from the school at Harriet Chapman Hospital. All but the last nurse in the row have been identified. They are: left to right – Gladys Melvin, Evelyn Cronkite, Frieda Mohler (married name Dowding), Bernice Bowman, and the unidentified graduate.

The nurses are sitting on the porch railing of the big porch at the hospital. Apparently they had not graduated yet because none of them is wearing a nurse's cap.

The brick wall at the left encloses the four-story elevator shaft. On the right is the large circular area with a wing extending around the corner. The entire porch was later enclosed for office space.

CHAPTER II

STIMSON HOSPITAL

The small proprietary hospital operating in Eaton Rapids was named STIMSON HOSPITAL, after Dr. Charles A. Stimson, M.D., who was the final survivor of the three people who had first founded it as the Harriet Chapman Hospital.

The Harriet Chapman Hospital had an excellent reputation. It had a recognized school of nursing, and graduated trained nurses each year. Dr. Stimson was a well-known proctologist, who needed the hospital to accommodate some of his patients, many of whom came long distances to consult him for anorectal problems, and to have surgery or other treatments. He often carried out complicated surgical procedures, and many of his patients required prolonged postoperative hospital care. Other doctors were allowed to use the hospital and also admitted patients. Stimson Hospital became a popular place in which to have a baby. Women living in the area rarely delivered at home. They came either to Stimson Hospital or to a comfortable maternity home operated by a registered nurse and located about a block away. The maternity home, however, had been closed for some time when I arrived in town. Dr. Stimson had also died before I came to town, and Bernice Bowman, the nurse who had operated the hospital for him, was running it. She had inherited half of it, and the doctor's widow, Mrs. Isabel Stimson, the other half, so the two women owned it together.

Small hospitals were not new to me, and I felt comfortable there. During my childhood, my uncle, Dr. Herman A. Meinke, M.D., established the Helene Meinke Hospital, named after his mother, my grandmother, in Hazel Park, Michigan. At the age of five years I had a Tonsillectomy and Adenoidectomy there, and later, at the age of fifteen, I had an appendectomy for a ruptured appendix in the very same operating room. Another uncle, Dr. Charles Kuhn, M.D., owned and operated a hospital near downtown Detroit named the Warren Diagnostic Hospital & Clinic. Small hospitals such as these, which were owned and operated by individuals, were known as proprietary hospitals.

On my first visit to Eaton Rapids Stimson Hospital was open and running with Bernice Bowman at the helm. I met her on my first visit there, and she took me on a tour of the hospital during which she explained much about how the hospital operated. As we went through I kept comparing it to my uncle's hospital, where I had not only been a patient, but had also participated from time to time in some of its operations by doing various needed chores, such as cleaning, painting and making minor repairs. I understood immediately what Stimson Hospital was and how it operated, and I felt comfortable about practicing there. My tour of the hospital with Bernice was what clinched my decision to come to Eaton Rapids to practice.

Eaton Rapids also offered some other favorable practice conditions. It was close to Lansing and Sparrow Hospital where I had interned, and to the University of Michigan Medical School from which I had received my medical degree. I would be able to comfortably turn to these two places for medical help if I should need it. I also chose Eaton Rapids as the town in which I would practice because I abhorred politics and political maneuvering, particularly medical politics. I thought, incorrectly, that if I practiced in a small town I would be essentially free of such activities.

The hospital building did not look like a hospital at all. Located on the corner of Main and Plain Streets, it still stands today. It was first used as a large residential dwelling, a mansion, so big that it took up most of the area of the city lot on which it stood. There wasn't even a sign outside to indicate its name or that it was a hospital. The main entrance had a half-flight of stairs up to the main entrance facing Plain Street. A second entrance in the back opened to a small porch, then down some stairs to the alley. The basement of the building was set quite shallowly into the ground, which exposed a considerable amount of basement wall above ground level. There were some large windows there, which allowed a lot of daylight into that part of the basement that was being used as the hospital kitchen.

Inside, just to the right of the back door entrance was an open stairwell, with staircases reversing direction at landings between the floors. It ran from the basement up to the third floor, and coming off of the landing between the second and third floor was a half-floor consisting of a hallway and two patient rooms. At the front of the building, directly opposite the stairway, was an elevator large enough to easily accommodate a hospital bed, and on all four floors (the basement included) a hallway ran the full length of the building from the stairs at one end to the elevator at the other.

With this arrangement it was not possible for the elevator to serve the half-floor, so it was necessary for patients using the hospital rooms there to negotiate a half-flight of stairs, up or down, in order to get to their beds. Bed-ridden patients assigned to those beds had to be carried, and this chore was facilitated by the use of a special stretcher (litter) that I believe was home made. It consisted of a stout piece of canvas about six feet long with wide lateral hems which were threaded on to stout wooden poles, both ends of which protruded a short distance beyond the canvas. This canvas was then evenly split in the middle, lengthwise, and wide hems were made in the new edges. These hems were then cut at about two inch intervals from their outer margins to, but not through, their sewed seams, and the cloth of every other two inch section was removed, so that when the two halves were placed together, the remaining sections could mesh together like gear teeth. The raw edges were finished (probably sewn by hand) to prevent raveling. Now a wide strap of harness leather was threaded through these alternating loops, which served to hold the two halves of the canvas stretcher securely together. A patient in surgery could be moved from the operating table to a gurney upon which this stretcher had been placed, wheeled to the head of the stairs, then easily carried by two strong people down the half-flight of stairs to the room, and placed on the bed. The leather strap would then be pulled from the stretcher while it was still under the patient, and the two halves could easily be separated and pulled away, one from each side.

Officially Stimson Hospital had thirteen hospital beds. None were on the main floor, where there was a large lobby, a small room used as a medical laboratory, a large, darkened room which housed a fairly new Picker x-ray machine, and some other spacious rooms which had been Dr. Stimson's offices and examination rooms. The basement below housed the hospital kitchen, some rooms for storing supplies, and a large dining room in which the staff usually ate.

The next floor above the lobby was the main floor of the hospital inpatient section. There were four beds in one large room that was used primarily as a maternity ward for new mothers. It was customary then for new mothers to be kept down in bed for ten days after their delivery, and at any given time there were usually some recently delivered new mothers in the hospital. There was also another ward-like room containing three beds, one room containing two beds, and two private rooms, all on the second floor. The two rooms on the in-between floor were private rooms.

The top floor also had its hallway running the full length of the building, with the stair shaft coming in at one end and the elevator shaft on the other. On the south side of the hall were the obstetrical delivery room and the newborn nursery. On the other side were the labor room and a large surgical operating room with a toilet and dressing room between them. The autoclave (sterilizer) and scrub sinks were not located in the hall but were in sort of an anteroom at the entrance to the surgery.

The newborn nursery had large windows facing the hall so that relatives could see the new babies without entering the room. The baby cribs were homemade, of wood, painted white. They looked something like tall bedside stands with a rail around the top, which kept the box built for the baby to sleep in from sliding off. The crib boxes contained mattress-like padding, and the babies had the usual baby blankets and garments. There were usually babies to be seen in the nursery, because post-partum mothers were being kept in bed for ten days after they delivered. This long hospital stay would soon be shortened because of the arrival of younger doctors and nurses coming back into practice from the War. It was rapidly becoming apparent that the long period of bed rest was actually detrimental to the newly delivered mother's health, and it was even believed to be the cause of some late post-partum hemorrhages and maternal vascular problems, such as venous thrombosis (clotting) and even sometimes-fatal emboli.

Because of those old-fashioned, long, hospital stays, the expected population of newly delivered mothers in the hospital at any one time was four. Often there were fewer, and sometimes there were more. There were extra cribs in the nursery for the babies, and the extra mothers were placed in other beds in the hospital when there was no longer space in the post partum maternity room. I recall that there was a time when the population of the hospital consisted of a post partum mother in every bed, all thirteen of them, and with so many obstetrical cases to care for, there arose a critical need for additional baby cribs in the nursery. Bernice solved this problem very nicely by going downtown to the A&P Store (a grocery store chain operated by the Great Atlantic & Pacific Tea Co.), where the manager gave her some of the big cardboard boxes in which bunches of bananas had arrived. With proper padding and additional baby bedding these made excellent cribs. Also, at this same time there was one additional patient in the hospital, --- a young man for whom I had removed an inflamed appendix. There was no place to put him after the operation, so he stayed overnight in the delivery room, until some of the obstetrical cases could be discharged.

The surgery had a high ceiling and appeared bright and airy because facing the North were four large windows, which did not open. They stretched from about four feet above the floor all of the way to the high ceiling, and let in a lot of light. They made up the entire wall opposite the door, and observed from the street below, looked something like a glass-enclosed widow's walk. After Stimson Hospital ceased operations and closed, the building stood idle for quite a while before it was remodeled into apartment dwelling units. Much later there was a fire on the top floor, which was badly burned. The top floor rooms were never rebuilt, but the top floor of the elevator shaft remained and was sealed off with a slanted portion of new roof, and a new roof was built over the second floor and the half-story which had contained the two private patient rooms. The building is still in use today as residential living quarters.

The Operating Room had a very adequate surgical floodlight in the ceiling, and there were two additional spotlights on movable stands to augment the ceiling light. There were no anesthesia machines. Open drop ether anesthesia with an ether mask was considered to be the safest anesthetic, and was the most widely used. Spinal anesthesia was also popular because of its relative simplicity and the superior muscle relaxation it produced. The usual surgical team consisted of a surgeon, an anesthetist, an assistant surgeon for major operations, a scrub nurse working in the sterile field, and a circulating nurse. Minor surgical operations were often done without a scrub nurse.

The labor room contained three beds and looked much like any of the other hospital rooms. When labor had proceeded to the verge of delivery the mother was taken across the hall to the delivery room. Sometimes when two women were about to deliver at nearly the same time, the operating table in the surgery was used for one of the deliveries. On rare occasions a patient had to be delivered in bed. Whenever it became necessary to do a Caesarian Section, it was done in the Operating Room.

The delivery room was primitive. A long, narrow room, it had only a dim ceiling light. A surgical spotlight on a movable stand was stationed at the foot of the delivery table, and provided the main illumination for whatever was being done. The delivery table was homemade, and consisted of two homemade, shallow, wooden boxes about three feet square and perhaps six inches deep. By themselves they looked like they might be sand boxes for children to play in. Turned up side down and fitted with iron pipe legs with flanges attached, they made two identical tables, which, when placed together, created a delivery table six feet long. Each half was padded with a thin mattress, and in the upper table, ----- the half upon which the mother's torso would rest, ----- large wooden blocks had been firmly fastened in two adjacent corners, and holes had been bored into them to accommodate stout steel rods which extended some distance above the mattress, then curved downward in a "U" shape. At the end of each there was a metal coupling which attached two loops of wide fabric strapping to it, one to support the mother's foot and the other her heel. With the long arm of the "U" inserted into the holes in the tabletop, and the mother's feet supported by the straps at the other end, these made up the stirrups used for delivery. When delivery was imminent, the mother's feet were put up into the loops and her torso was so positioned that her perineum did slightly overhang the division between the two tables. The lower table was then moved aside; sterile drapes were applied, and the doctor dressed in cap, mask, sterile gown and gloves would proceed with managing the delivery. The circulating nurse usually gave whatever anesthesia was given, which in the early days was usually open drop ether given with an ether mask. Almost never was it administered to the degree that the mother was rendered completely unconscious. In the amounts given the mother's senses would be dulled so that the pain was not felt so much. I think that because the ether smelled so terrible and had a tendency to cause choking and nausea, it had most of its effect in dulling the labor pains by taking the mother's mind away from them. There was no scrub nurse, so the doctor had the sterile field duties all to himself. The circulating nurse received the newborn baby in a sterile baby blanket.

For doing episiotomies, which are incisions made in the perineum to enlarge the external birth canal, local anesthesia by injection into the area of 1% procaine (Novocaine) worked very well, and allowed meticulous repairs to be done without pain. It also worked well for the repair of most tears (lacerations) sustained by the mother during the birth.

On the main floor of Stimson Hospital was a long, wide lobby with a floor of small white tiles running the full width of the building. On one side of it there were three office rooms, one of which had formerly been Dr. Stimson's office, and a short hallway to an exterior front door that opened to a porch. This porch went around the Northeast corner of the building, and exactly at the corner there was a large circular area with a diameter longer than the width of the porch, giving the appearance of a large, perfectly round bulge there. The porch was later enclosed, bulge and all, and heated to make additional medical examining rooms. The hallway on the other side of the lobby led past the X-ray room and a small medical laboratory across from it, which was located adjacent to the main stairwell, then ran past the stairwell to the back door. The laboratory was used by the nursing staff for doing simple tests such as urine sugar tests. The doctors did some of their own blood tests and a few other tests there, but no major laboratory tests were done. The mandatory serology tests for syphilis were routinely sent to the (Michigan) State Laboratory where they were done without charge.

The X-ray room had one window in it that was completely and permanently blocked out because the x-ray films that were exposed there were also developed there by hand. Complete darkness was required during the developing process, lest the films be ruined by exposure to light. We developed the X-ray films in a small alcove, where the processing tanks were located. A very small, dim red light, which emitted just enough red rays for the person developing the film to faintly see what he or she was doing, but not enough to spoil the film, was used during the developing process. The film was removed from its holder (cassette) in this otherwise total darkness, clamped into a special, stretcher-like metal frame, and put into a developer solution. Then when the developed picture appeared to be about right, it was transferred into a fixer solution. After the film had been in the fixer for a moment we could turn the regular lights back on again. Every film we exposed had to be developed in this manner.

There was a relatively new Picker X-ray machine with its x-ray tube enclosed in metal in the X-ray room. The tube, which produced the x-rays, was attached to a long arm, which could be moved parallel to the table top, and could be swung around at the head or the foot of the x-ray table to a position beneath it. With the tube in that position, the patient lying on the table, and the movable fluoroscope screen placed over the patient, fluoroscopy examinations were carried out. A drawback to this arrangement was that in order to take a good X-ray picture of an abnormality seen on the fluoroscopy screen, the tube had to be pulled out from under the table and the film had to be positioned under the patient, and also under the table, before the exposure could be made. In addition to moving the tube out from under the table, the fluoroscopy screen also had to be turned aside. In the time it took to accomplish all this, the abnormality that had been seen during fluoroscopy would most often have moved out of position, and the film would have missed it.

The table could be tilted up to a ninety-degree angle from the floor, and a patient on it could be viewed while in the upright position, which was the ideal position for watching the patient swallow a barium sulfate suspension to examine the esophagus, stomach and duodenum for ulcer and other diseases.

This brings to mind an examination I did, during those early days, upon a patient whose name escapes me now. He had given me a very good history for the diagnosis of duodenal ulcer, so I had scheduled an upper G.I. (Gastro Intestinal) examination. In those days we did our own examinations, and developed and read our own x-ray films. Bernice had mixed up the barium sulfate powder in milk, which was what we used as contrast material for this examination. For about fifteen minutes before we entered the darkened room we wore dark red goggles over our eyes to attenuate our pupils so we could more easily see the fluoroscopic images on the screen in the darkness. Without this preliminary procedure it would not be possible to immediately see the fluoroscopy images clearly, or to develop any x-ray films that might have been taken during an examination, until after our eyes had accommodated themselves to the pitch dark in the room.

Bernice had everything ready and assisted me. We placed the patient, wearing only a hospital gown, on the X-ray table, and, with the foot-platform attached to the table for him to stand upon, we tilted the table into the upright position to begin the examination. I gave the word to have the patient drink the usual milk and barium mixture. Watching the fluoroscope screen intently, I could see only a barely visible, faint shadow, which appeared to be passing down the esophagus. Something wasn't right! I thought that perhaps the patient was only gingerly sipping the mixture. I told him to take big swallows, and he promptly replied that he had already emptied the glass. I told Bernice that perhaps she had not made the mixture strong enough, and asked her to mix another glass "double strength." The patient drank most of this, but the results were no better. I was stumped. I had to call off the examination.

While the patient was dressing, I wondered what the problem had been, and was gathering my wits as to what I must tell him. Just then Bernice came to me with the answer. Barium sulfate, a white powder which we mixed into milk to make up the contrast material for these fluoroscopy examinations, was almost impervious to X-rays, and when an X-ray film was taken of a stomach full of this mixture, it kept the x-ray beams from reaching the film in the areas of its shadow. When developed the unaffected photographic emulsion would wash off, leaving this area blank. The shadow appeared white, in striking contrast to the developed film, and always appeared in the identical shape that the stomach had assumed when the film was exposed. Barium sulfate was least expensive when bought by the pound in bulk, and it came in large, barrel-shaped, waterproof containers made of heavy cardboard. This was the way we bought it. Likewise we bought Calcium sulfate in similar containers, and Bernice had mixed calcium sulfate instead of barium sulfate into the milk we had given to the patient.

The knowledge that calcium sulfate was **Plaster of Paris**, which we used for making hard plaster casts, and the knowledge that it would "set up" under water, like concrete, gave me a few anxious moments. I had visions of the Plaster of Paris hardening into a solid cast in the shape of the inside of the patient's stomach and duodenum, and almost immediately considered that such a problem could only be solved by surgically removing it. Then I thought that this probably would not happen because the properties which allowed the Plaster of Paris to set would be spoiled by the presence of stomach enzymes, acid and mucus. Additionally the stomach and duodenum were in almost constant motion, which would interfere with the setting process. From experience I knew that bending and reshaping the plaster in a cast while it was in the process of setting often caused it to weaken and crumble. I decided that the best course of action was to wait and see what would happen.

Of course I told the patient what had happened, assured him that calcium sulfate was not poisonous, and asked that he take some measures to avoid constipation. The antacid medication he was already taking had some of the properties of a laxative and, if taken in excessive dosages, could actually cause diarrhea, so I told him to continue taking it, and added a small dose of milk of magnesia (an excellent laxative) to be taken three times a day. He was to notify me in twenty-four hours if his bowels had not moved, to note the character of his stool for the next two or three days, and call me with this information.

It happened that the patient had no problems related to this incident. When he called me later, he told me that he had had several bowel movements and the only differences he noticed were that they were very light in color (Plaster of Paris is white.), and that the stool was coarse and grainy, filled with numerous particles like gravel or small pebbles. After that the patient's stomach problems seemed to be completely cured. At least he never complained about his stomach to me again.

There is a humorous sequel to this story. Some years later, while I was still practicing in my office in Stimson Hospital, our receptionist interrupted me as I was interviewing a patient, saying that there was a doctor in a small town North of us who wanted to speak to me. I excused myself, and went to a phone in another room. The following back and forth conversation ensued.

"Hello."

"Hello. Are you the doctor who gave Plaster of Paris to a patient during an upper G.I. exam?"

"Yes."

"What happened?"

"Nothing really. The patient passed it easily in the form of small plaster pellets."

"THANK GOD!!!!!"

"Click!"

The phone went dead.

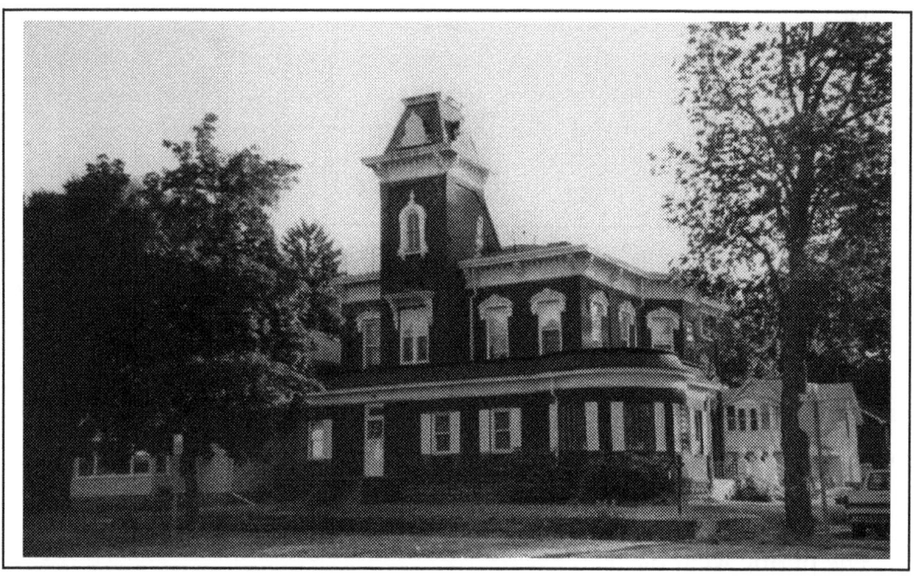

The Stimson Hospital building (formerly the Harriett Chapman Hospital) as it was in 2002. The fourth floor was destroyed by fire some time after the hospital closed. The damaged section was removed and a new roof was applied. The square section in front is the elevator shaft. The slanted roof behind it was necessary to cover the elevator door to the former fourth floor. The round area in the front (right) and the extensions were once a porch that was later enclosed to make medical offices and examining rooms. As seen in the picture there was no sign on the premises to show its name or to indicate that it was a hospital.

CHAPTER III

MY ARRIVAL IN TOWN

When I moved to Eaton Rapids in September of 1946 my wife was not able to come with me, because no new housing had been built there since before World War II, and there were no houses or apartments for rent. So we decided that she should stay with her parents in Detroit, at least until after the arrival of our first child, who was expected to be born sometime in December.

For temporary quarters I found a sleeping room to rent in a large old house on River Street, which was conveniently located between River Street and the Grand River, and was essentially just around the block from what would soon become my office downtown. The river at this location was approximately eighty feet wide, and in it there was a substantial island, which was perhaps forty feet wide and had been made into a city park. A sidewalk ran from River Street to a bridge that crossed one arm of the river, ran across the island, and then crossed another bridge to the other side of the river. One short block farther on, it reached Main Street, where the second store to the North from that corner was where my first office would be located. From the house we could see the river and the island, with its mounted Civil War cannons and a gazebo in which the city band occasionally played concerts in the summer. We could see the backs of some of the downtown stores.

The house was known as the **Webster House** because it had been built by the Webster family, and was still owned, by one of its well-known members. I rented my room from Ralph and Marian Berg, a middle aged couple who had rented the house from the Websters, and were subletting sleeping rooms to help make ends meet. Marian did the housekeeping, shopped for groceries, cooked, and also had a part-time job in a grocery store downtown. Ralph was an oil and lubricant salesman who called upon farm people to sell his wares. Shortly after I moved in, Mrs. Berg offered board in addition to the room, and I arranged to have evening meals there. I found Mrs. Berg's cooking far more satisfying than the restaurant food I had been eating.

Two other roomer/boarders were also living there,------- Miss Esma Ferguson, a high school teacher, who later taught my children in school, and remained a good friend throughout the rest of her life, and another teacher who didn't stay in Eaton Rapids very long, ------- a younger blonde woman whose name I can't remember.

The house was typical of the old-fashioned mansions that well-to-do people had built in past generations. Constructed of wood, there was a large porch on the North side of the house from which the main entrance opened into a large living room. The main floor also included a large dining room, a pantry, and a country kitchen large enough to comfortably hold the large dining table at which we ate most of our evening meals. There was a bathroom between the kitchen and a large master bedroom located at the front of the house, and from that bedroom a door opened into the living room. Opposite the main door into the house, between the living room and dining room, an open stairway led to an upstairs hall, which provided access into several bedrooms and an unusually large bathroom. There was also a basement with a furnace that was fed by a coal stoker.

My first day of work, near the end of August 1946, began in the afternoon in Dr. VanKolken's office, which was located near the north end of Main Street. Dr. Van Kolken was not there, but physical examinations for football players and other high school athletes had been scheduled for me. I arrived soon after lunch, and Mary Van Auker, the office assistant-receptionist, mistook me for one of the high school football players, pointed to a door and said, "Go in there, and strip to the waist." Such a mistake was not exactly a rarity in those days. Although I was almost twenty-seven years old, I believe I looked younger. Mary was embarrassed when I introduced myself and told her who I was.

The physical examinations went well. I examined a lot of healthy high school boys. There were no signs of serious illness, but I was impressed by the generally poor teeth that these young people had. An occasional one in this group had already lost all of his teeth, and I assumed that it was from decay, because many of these aspiring athletes had dental cavities. I did not charge anything for these examinations, and in all of my years of practice I never did charge for any of the school athletic physicals that I did. To the best of my knowledge, neither did the other doctors in town. I also saw a few regular patients that afternoon, and enjoyed the experience. I concluded afterward that to stay and practice in this small town would be just fine. The people seemed to have complaints of a kind that I was expecting, and I was comfortable with discussing their problems and prescribing treatment. Besides, I planned to practice only a few years, save up enough money, to enter a surgical residency somewhere, and become a board certified surgeon, but in the end my wife and I found the people of Eaton Rapids to be so nice and so friendly that we never did leave.

While I was serving my abbreviated (nine months – November 1943 through July 1944) internship at Sparrow Hospital in Lansing, World

War II was at its height, and there was a noticeable scarcity of doctors all over Southern Michigan. At that time Sparrow Hospital had five floors with more than 300 beds, but had only three interns for most of the time that I was there. Each of us had to cover the emergency service for twenty-four hours every second or third day. Once the staff physicians recognized that we had been decently educated, we were left much on our own to treat emergency room patients, and refer them for follow-up to their doctor's office. We treated illnesses, sprains and strains, set minor fractures and applied casts, and repaired almost all of the cuts and lacerations that could be sewed up under local anesthesia. When emergency room patients required hospital admission, we admitted them for the staff doctor of their choice. During the War those doctors who were left behind to practice seemed to be happy to have us do these things, because they were generally overworked and chronically tired.

These circumstances provided me with many extraordinary opportunities for doing procedures and operations (under supervision at first), which I would not otherwise have had. Most of the obstetricians allowed me to deliver babies for them, and after only a very short time allowed me to repair episiotomy incisions. Soon I was doing these things by myself, and felt highly flattered that some doctors regularly trusted me with doing the repairs after they had delivered the baby. Working as a battalion surgeon at the battlefront in Italy during the War had also exposed me to enough shattered bones and open wounds, so that I had long since lost any squeamishness that I may have had over the sight of blood.

As I started to practice in Eaton Rapids, I suddenly realized that I had already had more "hands-on" surgical experience than most general practitioners of that era. Indeed, I felt confident that I was well able to handle a general practice, and could comfortably meet the needs of the people in and around Eaton Rapids. I believed that I was able to do more for them than the average family physician. Before long I began to consider my patients a bit as if they were my extended family, and I was happy with my feeling of belonging, a feeling which reinforced my determination to, above all, do no harm to anyone.

Although I never did leave to take a residency, I did gradually work myself into a large surgical practice, and I believe that I did become a good surgeon. This was accomplished by continuing with "book-learning" from surgical textbooks and journals, and by working with, and assisting good surgeons as often as possible. As long as I was in practice, I never stopped learning. At first I scrubbed in as often as I could with Dr. Ralph Wadley, M.D, a most prolific, top-notch surgeon from Lansing, who came to Eaton Rapids to consult and operate whenever he was needed. I also occasionally provided anesthesia for him, particularly when scheduling circumstances dictated that he had to operate upon one of my patients in Sparrow or St.

Lawrence Hospital in Lansing. I also learned much from the obstetrician, Dr. Jason Meads, M.D. of Jackson, who performed caesarian sections in Stimson Hospital for me before I started doing them myself. He came to Eaton Rapids whenever he was needed to consult on a complicated delivery. He was an expert in what was called "version and extraction", an obstetrical manipulation in which, after the uterine cervix was fully dilated, he reached in, turned the baby end for end, and delivered it as a breech extraction. I saw him do this a number of times, but was always wary of doing it myself, because a newborn baby's head is the body part which has the largest diameter, and to be unable to quickly get it out of the birth canal, once the body was born, would mean that the baby would die of suffocation. Later I learned more surgery from my brother, Richard K. Meinke, M.D. who received his excellent surgical training at the Mayo Clinic in Rochester, Minnesota, then came to Lansing to practice. Later I learned much from my son, Albert H. Meinke, III, M.D., who served his surgical residency at the University of Kentucky in Lexington, and came to practice for a while in Eaton Rapids.

CHAPTER IV

MY FIRST OFFICE

During that first afternoon of practice in Dr. VanKolken's office I learned that I would not be able to rent his space as my office. His lease was ending, and the owner of the building had plans to remodel it for a different use. This forced me to look for other suitable, rentable, medical office space, and I engaged Roy Heminger of Heminger's Real Estate, a business on Main Street run by Roy and Vera Heminger, to help me find it. The Hemingers seemed to make a good team. Roy was the salesperson, and Vera did the paperwork. Before long Roy reported to me that the only rentable space downtown was a barbershop, which had gone out of business, which had been known as Gunnell's Barber Shop. All of its furnishings and fixtures remained inside, and as a condition of renting the space I was obliged to buy everything there. There appeared to be no other practical alternative, so I agreed, and rented it by the month.

The space available was about the same as that in most of the smaller retail stores on Main Street. Included in the furnishings were two standard barber chairs that were in working order, six or eight high backed wooden chairs, and some knick-knacks and bric-a-brac. I could use some of the waiting room chairs, and there was a basement into which I could put most of the rest of it. The barber chairs were large, heavy, and difficult to move, so I advertised them for sale, and managed to sell the one that was in the best condition for ten dollars. Finally I had to pay someone to haul the other one to the local trash dump.

After I had emptied it completely, I found that I had rented what was essentially a store with a high ceiling and a large, storefront window facing on Main Street. Alterations were needed to turn it into something resembling a doctor's office. The entrance door at the South front corner of this room was set at a forty five degree angle to the street in order to allow space for an alcove outside from which another door, placed parallel to the street, opened upon a stairway leading to offices upstairs. Underneath these stairs were the stairs that descended from my rented area into my basement. There was no back door to outside.

The work of remodeling was not complicated, and I did it myself. I installed a substantial curtain to cover the big plate glass store window and shield my waiting room from the vision of curious people on the street. I did the carpentry myself. Plywood paneling nailed on to two by four frames enclosed the rear two thirds of the space to form two examining rooms. This left the front of the store to be the waiting room in which I placed a reception desk with telephone where Mary VanAuker made appointments, handled patients, and kept the books for my practice. She also assisted and protected me, when necessary, during examinations. I also bought Dr. VanKolken's medical equipment, which, besides medicines and medical instruments, included a cot and a standard examining table with stirrups. The examining table plus my small desk and two visitor chairs were put into the larger office, and the cot went into the small examining room. The passageway created by the construction of these rooms was used as a hallway to get into them from the waiting room, and on the opposite side of it was the door that led downstairs to the basement. The farthermost back of this hallway became a "dead" end into which I built a counter and shelves for holding my microscope, medicines to be dispensed, a centrifuge, and some other laboratory equipment that I intended to use in my office. There was also a sterilizer used for sterilizing medical instruments and minor surgical tools.

Mine was probably the crudest, most crowded office of any doctor in the county, but I felt that under the circumstances it was the most practical arrangement I could have in order to begin practice without going deeply into debt. However, I was not able to avoid debt entirely. To do the remodeling and other things required in order to begin my practice I needed more money than I had available, so I applied for a loan at the local bank, which was then the National Bank of Eaton Rapids. After I had pledged all of my office equipment as collateral and had my father co-sign the note, the bank let me have $1,500. This seemed to me to be an enormous debt at the time, but my practice was able to repay it, with interest, on schedule.

Mrs. Mary VanAuker, who had been Dr. VanKolken's receptionist-bookkeeper-medical assistant agreed to come to work for me, and she was of great help by introducing me to many people in the area. I needed malpractice insurance and took out a policy with the Medical Protective Company. As I can best recall that first year's premium was in the neighborhood of seventy dollars, a sharp contrast to the thousands of dollars I paid for such insurance coverage in the latter years of practice. As a requirement needed to be able to buy the insurance I had to belong to the local and state medical societies, so I joined the Eaton County Medical Society, the Michigan State Medical Society, and the American Medical Association. In those early years the dues I paid to those organizations were modest, but they too have increased tremendously with the passage of time. I also engaged an accounting and consulting service named Professional Management with headquarters in Battle Creek, Michigan, to set up my accounting system, begin the accounting, and send someone to my office once per month to audit my books. They also prepared my income tax returns at the end of each year, and from time to time advised me of necessary and desirable changes in the way I carried on my practice. Professional Management continued in this role later on for the professional corporation in which I practiced, but by then I was using a different certified public accounting firm to prepare my income tax returns.

CHAPTER V

MY PRACTICE BEGINS

Office Call - $3.00; House Call – $5.00; Obstetrical Case (Prenatal office visits, Delivery and Hospital Care, plus a six week checkup) - $30.00; Appendectomy including pre and postoperative care - $75.00. These are examples of my charges when I began to practice, and they were typical of what most general practitioners in the area charged. I remember that on Thursday afternoon during my first week only two patients came in for office visits, and I suffered a bit of uneasiness as to whether or not I would make a go of it.

Although my practice began slowly, it grew steadily. In retrospect I now realize that I was doing a number of things that practically guaranteed my success. I kept better than average medical records for those times. My patients watched me do it, and knew I was doing it. For keeping patients' clinical records I used full-page sized folders and the medical forms, recommended and furnished by Professional Management. Patients seemed surprised that I regularly did such things as urinalyses, checked hemoglobin levels, and occasionally did blood counts in my office, and I didn't charge extra for doing these things. I also did not charge for doing the "Well Baby Examinations," when mothers brought their children in for immunizations, and because the State Health Department Laboratory provided the vaccines free of charge, I did not charge for them either. I did charge a small fee to cover the costs of the needles and syringes used to administer the shots. I believe that all of these things helped my practice grow rapidly, and later, after I had become very busy, I did not have the heart to change these policies.

Although there were three drug stores with pharmacies in town, I found it necessary to dispense medicines. The drug stores were all located in the same block on Main Street, -----**Milbourne's** on one side, and **Shimmin's** and **Heaton's** on the other. Each was owned and operated by a pharmacist by the same name. Although the drug stores closed daily at 5:00 or 6:00 PM, and were normally closed on Sunday, all three druggists told me to call them if I had an emergency need for some medication. I did call, but not often. There were plenty of minor emergencies and pseudo-emergencies during the hours when the drug stores were closed. Most were not life threatening, or likely to result in permanent disability, so generally I did not disturb the druggists for such cases.

However, I soon learned that patients were much more satisfied if they were able to start their medications immediately, so I carried a lot of medicines in my office and in the bag that I took with me on house calls. This enabled me to supply on-the-spot starter doses to my patients. I kept injectable medications in my office, and carried some in my medical bag. In my bag I also carried pain relievers, tranquilizers, antacids and digestants, digitalis, diuretics, drugs for asthmatics, anticonvulsants, and several kinds of narcotics, which meant that I had to have a current narcotics license and keep complete and precise records of all narcotics which passed through my hands. I did not charge extra beyond the charge for the house call or office call for dispensing single injections or small amounts of medicines as starter doses.

The three drug stores in town were eager to furnish prescription pads for me, so I was amply supplied. In the early days I also bought some medicines at these drug stores to replenish what I usually carried in my medical bag.

Many folk medicines were in use in the area, and I gradually learned about most of them. I quickly learned that an ointment named "Bag Balm," which was for sale to treat the teats of milk cows for various inflammations, was very popular as an all-purpose salve, which human beings in the area seemed to be using freely. Some women told me that they used it on their own nipples during pregnancy and while nursing their babies in order to "toughen them up". Various poultices and "plasters" were in common use, and were made with a wide variety of materials including mustard, onions, peppermint, wood ashes, and well rotted manure. In the surrounding farmlands were a number of areas of muck land, where the soil was usually wet and very black. This made it excellent for raising garden vegetables and herbs. Peppermint was a popular crop, and was grown in large muck fields. Those farmers who had their own stills could distill their harvest right in the field to collect the peppermint oil, which was the product that was sold. These farmers would also, for a fee, distill the peppermint crops of area farmers who did not have their own still.

A wide variety of herbal remedies, mostly in the form of teas steeped from dried leaves or roots, were also popular. One of the herbal laxatives used by a large number of people had for years been promoted by Dr. Stimson, who dispensed it from his Stimson Hospital office. After he died, his widow and Bernice Bowman continued to produce the product and sell it to the public. They were still doing a brisk business years after Dr. Stimson was gone, and people were still coming long distances to the hospital to buy it. Convenient to the production of this remedy was the local dairy, **Miller Dairy Farms**, which was well known for its good ice cream. Miller Dairy Farms had its own large herds of milk cows, which were cared for and milked on satellite farms in the area. Since its main retail products were ice creams, the skim milk that was left over was normally available. It was dehydrated and sold as powdered skim milk. Dr. Stimson bought powdered skim milk, laced it with senna powder, a laxative that tends to promote liquid or soft stools. He then packed the finished product into round, one-pint sized ice cream cartons with directions as to how much of it should be taken daily, and sold them to the public.

My office had not been open very long before I learned about drug detail men. They acted as agents for the various drug companies to promote their products. When they came to call, they provided useful information about their various drug products, provided literature and samples, and often left advertising items for their products such as paperweights, rulers, mechanical pencils and pens, etc. Most of the time I had trouble remembering the names of these people, so I soon gave up trying. However, I usually could remember the name of the drug company for which they worked, so I would call them by their company name: --- Mr. Lilly, Mr. Parke-Davis, Mr. Ciba-Geigy, etc. There were then a lot of drug companies and medical supply houses that were not well known, which in the aggregate supplied thousands of kinds of pills, capsules and other medicines, many of which contained multiple drugs. I bought and carried some of them to dispense. I could often achieve the same desired medical effect in a patient, who was losing faith in his prescribed medication, by prescribing another pill with a similar mix of contents. The excellent effect of this maneuver on the patient's health and well-being often surprised me.

This phenomenon is known in medicine as "the placebo effect," and in the early years of my medical practice it was very useful, because the patient, convinced that the treatment was effective, would feel much better, and in many cases would actually get over his infections or heal his wounds faster because of it.

Although I am sure that the placebo effect exists unchanged today, I also know that our government has decimated its effect in the practice of medicine. First the Federal Drug Administration made it illegal to administer mixtures of drugs in a single pill or capsule. Next the "safety" and "efficacy (effectiveness)" of single drugs needed to be "proven" before the drug could be prescribed, and finally an approved drug could only be prescribed for certain, specific diagnoses or conditions. The final blow to the usefulness of placebos came from the medical insurance companies, especially those that sold "Prescription Insurance." To write a prescription for a placebo is now completely futile. The secret would be gone, and to think that the government or insurance company will pay for any substance labeled as a placebo is purely wishful thinking.

Nevertheless, the placebo effect is definitely still intact, hale and hearty. Only its usefulness in treating illness has drastically diminished. Doctors regularly read through long treatises covering the side effects of the drugs they prescribe, and in almost every study in which the effects of the drug in question is compared to a placebo, there are one or more categories of symptoms, such as nausea or diarrhea, which occur in greater numbers among those taking the sugar pills than in those taking the drug. The placebo effect is alive and well in so called holistic medicine, herbal medicine, manipulative medicine, voodoo, primitive medicines and outright quackery. This is attested by the millions of people, world wide, who pay money measured in billions of dollars per year for such medicines and treatments. No scientific evidence exists to show that they actually work. Their effect is a true placebo effect. People feel better because they truly believe that whatever they are taking or doing will improve their health and well-being. In some cases the placebo effect may help the patient feel better while nature heals the real disease that he has. The placebo effect exists! What rational being would pay for treatment or medicine over and over again, unless it truly made him feel better?

Another sphere of activity in which the placebo effect is alive and flourishing is in religion. Early in his anthropological development prehistoric man developed spoken language, and became able to communicate readily between individuals. With language came a primitive ability to reason, and, with reasoning, man became able to think about and understand the many real dangers in life that he faced. Eventually, without actually facing one of them at the moment, he could know that there were wild animals out in the field and forest that wanted to kill him and eat him. He could comprehend and understand other things which threatened him, such as storms with lightning and thunder, the danger of falling long distances, the danger of being caught alone in the territory of an enemy tribe, etc. Eventually, he even became able to imagine all manner of goblins and spooks ready to pounce on him and do him all kinds of harm, and in this manner mankind evolved into a life filled with fears. Early in the development of this "fearful life" the concept of protective deities entered his mind. Thus, religion for mankind was born.

Since the first group of early humans established their gods and their icons to worship, humans have developed literally thousands of religions. Religion didn't just happen. It was developed by people, because there was a universal need for it to alleviate and mitigate their large number of fears that had developed in men's minds, and had become a part of their daily lives. Some religions were simple, and we have archaeological evidence that some were very complex. Whether they worshipped one god or many, whether its rites and ceremonies were simple or extremely elaborate, and no matter what beliefs were embraced, each religion was born out of mankind's need for religion, and its purpose was to protect the individual from his fears and the mental anguish that his fears engendered.

What all religions do for their followers is to partially or completely relieve their anxieties and fears. They do so by prescribing rituals and beliefs, which may have little or no foundation in scientific data, but must be taken on faith. Those who believe, feel better. Their anxiety decreases. The fear of death is lessened. All of such accomplishments are perfect examples of the "placebo effect."

In my early days many of the medicines and the way they were used in and around Eaton Rapids seemed odd and behind the times to me. I knew very little of the practices of Dr. Hargrave and Dr. Irwin except for what patients and friends told me. I only remember meeting Dr. Hargrave once in Heaton's Drug Store, and concluded that he was a knowledgeable doctor. At the time he was not practicing very much any more, and spent a lot of time out of town at his property in the Upper Peninsula of Michigan. Not long after our conversation he became very ill with what was rumored to be a blood disease, which rendered him a "bleeder," and shortly thereafter he was admitted to a Lansing hospital where he died.

My first conversation with Dr. Irwin came only about three weeks after I had started practice. He called me on the phone and asked if I would make a house call to consult on one of his patients. He told me over the phone that he had been treating this man with Aconite, Byronium and Gelsemium, but the patient had not responded, and for days had been going downhill. I agreed to go, but first I had to look up to find out what these medicines were that he had prescribed. I already knew that Gelsemium was an herbal preparation, which had mild tranquilizing or sleep producing effects, but I knew nothing about the other two. I learned that they were also herbals, and that their effects were weak or doubtful.

When I arrived at the patient's house he was semi-comatose and could not be aroused enough to obtain any history of his illness from him. His family told me that he had been complaining of severe headaches, and more recently of nausea. They also volunteered that he had "not been himself" for six or eight months, and when I asked some leading questions they agreed that he had displayed a definite personality change. I suspected a brain problem immediately, and began to check reflexes, ability to move, and responses to sensory stimuli. Then, when I examined his eye grounds with my opthalmoscope, the diagnosis sprang out at me. He had papilledema, a bulging outward of the optic disks into the posterior chamber of the eye. The optic disks are the visible ends of the optic nerves, and are located at the back of the posterior chamber of the eyeball. This was papilledema of such a severe degree, as I had never before seen. It is caused by a sharp increase in the cerebrospinal fluid pressure within the skull, and when severe it often means brain tumor. I called Dr. Irwin back, told him what I thought, and said that I would try to get his patient into the hands of a neurosurgeon. Dr. Irwin agreed, saying that he was glad to be rid of the case. That afternoon I managed to arrange for the patient's admission to a hospital in Battle Creek, Michigan, and sent him there by ambulance. The next evening the neurosurgeon phoned me to say that the patient had died of his huge brain tumor before any operation could be done.

Several patients told me another interesting story about Dr. Irwin's office practice. It seems that he had a glass-enclosed cabinet in his office, of the type seen in many barbershops of those times. In it there was a strong ultra violet light. Barbers kept their scissors, clippers and razors, etc. in it with the presumption that the ultra violet light would sterilize them. Although ultraviolet light is capable of killing microbes and other living cells, there are all kinds of nooks and crannies in most instruments where it is not possible for the light rays to reach, and these instruments could not possibly be made surgically sterile in this manner.

A treatment prescribed by Dr. Irwin was to take a blood sample from a patient's arm vein, put it into a small glass tube, and store it under the ultraviolet light in the cabinet overnight. The patient would then return the next day, to have his own blood returned to him by intramuscular injection into the buttock. Now this is not as ridiculous a treatment as it might at first appear to be. Subtle changes would certainly occur in the blood sample by just being out of the body overnight, and changes caused by exposure to the ultraviolet light must also occur. When the blood is reinjected into the patient it would most likely behave somewhat like a foreign protein injection. In those days, injections of certain foreign proteins were commonly used to stimulate antibody production and hopefully increase the patient's immunity to infections. The real misgivings that these patients had was that the doctor was getting so old and infirm that they could not be completely sure that they were getting their own blood back.

Although Dr. Irwin continued his office practice, I cannot remember that he ever had a patient in Stimson Hospital. I do not remember seeing him or carrying on a conversation with him for over ten years, until he became my patient in the Eaton Rapids Community Hospital shortly after it opened. He was then well advanced in age, and died during that admission of congestive heart failure.

The first time I met Dr. Kraft of Leslie, Michigan he asked me to travel the rural area in which he practiced to give open drop ether anesthetics at ten dollars each to children in the farm homes, while he removed their tonsils and adenoids, a procedure called a T&A. He said that he usually did these with the patient lying on a table in the kitchen of the farmhouse. I declined this offer for several reasons. The main one was that I did not consider T&A to be a minor procedure, and I believed that it was much safer to do it in a hospital operating room. Because it was then a common operation, I had studied the technique thoroughly, and during my internship had done several T&As under supervision. For a long time during my early practice years, while doing one, I would wonder who the first doctor to do such an operation might have been. I believed that he must have been fearless or perhaps reckless, because during the proper removal of tonsils and adenoids there is always much bleeding, and the entire operative field is deep in the throat and difficult to see. Exposure of the tonsillar arteries in order to tie them off and stop their bleeding is always difficult. And not far away in the neck are the large blood vessels, which if punctured or severed could result in a major calamity. The posterior capsule of each tonsil is only a pinch of tissue away from the corresponding main carotid artery in the neck, and if a carotid artery were to be seriously injured, or severed, the bleeding would be horrendous and the situation would probably result in a fatality.

Properly removing a tonsil and its capsule from its bed in the side of the back of the throat requires sharp knife incisions for the full length of the tonsil pillars, where the tonsils are attached to the mucous membrane of the throat, and then blunt dissection to separate the tonsil and its capsule from its bed. The removal of the tonsil is usually completed by using a wire tonsil snare, which can be made to bluntly dissect away from its bed, any remaining tonsil capsule still clinging to it, and finally to sever the attachment at the lower pole. This then leaves a relatively large cavity in the throat where the tonsil had been, and leaves the two main tonsillar arteries stretched, severed, dangling and often bleeding. Space limitation in the mouth and throat make it difficult to clamp these arteries and tie them off. Control of bleeding usually begins by holding gauze, shaped into a tonsil-sized ball, pressed against the raw area. There are ring-ended clamps specially made for this purpose. They look like elongated hemostats, which have been bent into a "U" shape, but with small rings at the tips. The clamp holds the gauze ball in the tonsil cavity while the rest of the instrument dangles out of the way out of the corner of the mouth. With this in place the tonsil bed is "packed," and the bleeding is at least temporarily stopped. The tonsil on the opposite side is then removed in the same fashion.

The gauze packs are usually left in place long enough for the patient's blood coagulation system to "clot off" the open ends of the severed vessels, and sometimes, when they are removed, the bleeding seems to be well controlled. If bleeding continues or reoccurs, it is usually from one of the tonsillar arteries, which must then be clamped off, and tied, or sewed shut with suture material.

Adenoids are masses of lymphatic tissue growing in the back of the throat, behind the nose, and when there is very much of it present, it interferes with normal nasal breathing, and sometimes interferes with free drainage of the middle ear cavity through the eustachian tubes. Adenoid tissue is removed with an instrument called an adenotome and/or with adenoid curettes. The working part of an adenotome consists of a curved guide, which controls the direction of thrust of a wide flat blade, which does the cutting of the adenoid tissue. This guide is shaped to approximate the curve of the posterior nasopharynx, and slots along its sides guide the cutting blade through this curve as the blade is pushed forward. The blade itself is very thin and flexes easily to follow the guide slots. The cutting edge then neatly severs any adenoid tissue growing there. The handle of the adenotome is so curved as to make it easy to place this guide portion up behind the soft palate against the back of the nasaopharynx. When so placed with the blade retracted, much of the adenoid tissue present is pushed into the central area of the guide and held there. The blade is then pushed forward and the tissue amputated in much the same manner as a guillotine severed the necks of the unfortunate during the French Revolution.

This maneuver usually removes most but not always all of the adenoid tissue present, so the next step is to scrape away as much of any remaining adenoid tissue as possible with an adenoid curette, which is an instrument with one end having a curved frame. It is shaped to somewhat resemble a garden hoe, except that the adenoid curette blade is a more or less square frame with a cutting edge facing the inside of the square at its far end. It is placed on the back of the throat, pushed upward behind the soft palate as far as possible, pressed against the back wall of the nasopharynx, then swept downward across it to scrape off any remaining adenoid tissue.

This procedure is also usually accompanied by a lot of bleeding, and large, raw areas remain after the adenoid tissue is gone. Control of the bleeding usually begins with pressure applied in the form of gauze sponge "balls" and/or other gauze packing, which must be kept in place long enough for the patient's natural blood coagulation processes to come in to play and stop the bleeding. About ten minutes is usually sufficient. Occasionally the denuded adenoid area will continue to bleed and must to be packed with gauze held in place with tapes through each nostril with a third tape, to be used later to remove the packing, coming out through the mouth. These packs are customarily left in place overnight.

Later on, after we had the equipment to do electrocoagulation, we could clamp each individual tonsillar artery with a long tonsil hemostat, and then touch the hemostat with the coagulating electrode for a second to coagulate it. The smaller vessels could be coagulated directly by touching them with the same electrode. As each small vessel was "burned" the bleeding from it stopped abruptly, and when all had been treated this way the operative sites were "dry."

At first I was elated with this procedure, and thought that all of our bleeding problems had been solved. But not so. After I had begun using this method of hemostasis for a time, it became too often necessary to take a patient back into the operating room to stop the late bleeding which occurred, usually in the middle of the night after the operation, when the coagulum which had originally stopped the bleeding from one of the tonsillar arteries sloughed out. Then, with the patient once more under general anesthesia, I had to ligate (tie off) the bleeding vessel. These bleeders were difficult to stop because the end of the artery had been heated and burned, and there was not much artery left to identify. The bleeding often appeared to be coming from a hole in the wall of the cavity left behind after removal of the tonsil. To stop it was often difficult, and I often had to place a catgut suture (stitch) into the tissues in order to stop the bleeding. I soon stopped using electrocoagulation of the tonsillar arteries. There are two on each side, inferior and superior, and I began to routinely tie them off during the T&A operation, but continued to use cautery on minor bleeders, because this definitely shortened the total operating time and decreased blood loss. This practice stopped the late postoperative bleeding, and solved the problem.

In those days tonsils which were removed were generally either chronically infected or excessively large. The large ones interfered with drainage of the middle ear through the eustachean tubes, and often contributed to recurring middle ear infections and earaches. The chronically infected ones gave rise to recurrent sore throats. Many showed dried up pus in their crypts, and I, for one, felt that if any of the bacteria they harbored were streptococci, they were contributing to the high incidence of rheumatic fever and rheumatic heart disease that we were encountering in our practice. A number of patients with bad tonsils had had peritonsillar abscesses, which are serious infections with an accumulation of pus under the tonsil capsule. These often required incision and drainage, or they would rupture and drain spontaneously. After the drainage, tonsillectomy was usually deferred until after the tissue swelling had receded and the abscess walls had turned into scar tissue. The presence of such scar tissue, and any residual swelling made the dissection to free the tonsil capsule from its attachments to the deeper neck tissues more difficult and risky. Occasionally we read about a child dying during or shortly after a tonsillectomy. I remember that it occurred once during my internship at Sparrow Hospital, and although I was not involved with the surgery, I believe it was a case with complications as I have just described.

For many years after World War I tonsillectomy and adenoidectomy (T & A) was a very common operation, but after penicillin and other later antibiotics came into use the operation gradually lost favor. I believe that this came about because acute tonsillitis was generally treated and relatively quickly cured with antibiotics, preventing the development of so-called chronic tonsillitis. Competent surgeons did the tonsillectomies in excellent fashion, but even they, occasionally left a bit of tonsil capsule behind. The poorer surgeons of the day often left varying amounts of tonsil capsule behind. I believe that many times the tonsil capsule was not completely dissected free, and the tonsil snare could only cut through the tonsil somewhere above the capsule.

There was also another method of doing a tonsillectomy in which an instrument called a tonsillotome was used. This instrument consisted of a large metal ring across which a thin, flat blade could be shoved to cut through any tissue, encircled by the ring, in guillotine fashion, similar to the adenotome, which I have previously described. In order to use it, the tonsil could not be "buried" behind the tonsil pillars, but had to protrude toward the middle of the pharynx, as some did. In these cases the ring was placed over the tonsil, and the tonsil was pushed through it as far as was easily possible and fixed there with a fork like apparatus that speared the portion of tonsil that protruded and was to be removed. When the blade was pushed home it would take off a lot of tonsil tissue but would often leave much or all of the tonsil capsule behind. In these cases the tonsils invariably "grew back," and in those days this seemed to be a common occurrence. That wasn't all bad, however. Most of the patients who had had this done could breathe much more easily after the surgery. Many ceased having one recurrent infection after another, and because tonsil and adenoid tissue regresses with age, even the incomplete removal of tonsils eventually resulted in a permanent cure. I have examined many "oldsters," who had never had tonsils and adenoids removed, in which I could not find any recognizable tonsil or adenoid tissue. Most of the people who had had only "partial" tonsillectomies had their remaining tonsil and adenoid tissue regress in the same way.

Today, I still believe that a kitchen table in a farmhouse is no place to do a T&A!

Once begun it did not take long for my medical practice to become busy. Mary VanAuker was well known in the area, and I am sure that, because she worked for me, many of her friends and acquaintances came to me as patients. Dr. VanKolken had given me the list of obstetrical patients who had been coming to him for prenatal care before he left Eaton Rapids, and most of them remained with me for their deliveries. I soon delivered my first baby in Stimson Hospital, a boy born to a Mrs. Edick, who lived on a farm some miles to the West toward Charlotte, Michigan. Some fifty-five years later I had the pleasure of meeting this baby again when he was a teacher in the Eaton Rapids High School. Babies that Dr. VanKolken had delivered were also being brought to me for immunizations and general childhood care.

My wife, Edmere, was due to deliver our first child in late December. She remained in Detroit, where she lived with her parents, and was receiving her prenatal care in nearby Highland Park. I was living on River Street in the Webster House where I roomed and boarded with Ralph and Marian Berg. The Bergs were most accommodating people, allowing me, among other things, to receive phone calls for my new practice on their phone, and even taking requests for house calls for me when I was out. Although Mrs. Berg had a job in a downtown grocery store, she offered her roomers the evening meal, as a "room and board" service, and all of the roomers accepted. We usually all ate together at the big kitchen table, and I distinctly remember that the food was much better than the restaurant food I had been eating.

It became my routine to see my hospital patients each morning and do scheduled minor surgery either there or in my office. Then in the afternoons I would hold office hours, and afterward make house calls both before and after supper. Emergencies were dealt with over the phone during which the decision would be made to meet with the patient somewhere. Ambulance services were supplied by the local funeral directors, usually at five dollars per trip, with the driver and a second man in attendance.

My "Doctor Bag"--- the bag which I took with me on house calls was big and heavy, and contained many more things than most people might imagine would be in it. I carried two leather cases filled with glass vials, sixteen of them with screw caps, from which I dispensed a variety of pills and capsules, including narcotics, digitalis preparations, various hypnotics and sleeping pills, atropine, ergotrate, ephedrine, etc. I also carried five or six larger glass containers from which I dispensed such things as antacids and other preparations for treating unsettled stomachs, analgesics including aspirin and other combinations, and a number of sulfonamides to use against infections. I also carried syringes and hypodermic needles, and a variety of injectables, which included penicillin, several stimulants, several hypnotics, two injectable narcotics (morphine and Demerol), injectable digitalis, injectable liver extract, injectable hormones (estrogens, androgens, pituitrin), ergotamine for uterine bleeding, vitamin K for bleeding problems, and other preparations. For many years I carried a can of ether and an ether mask, and was happy to find that it was there when I needed it to break up a severe asthma attack in a young, teenaged girl after all other medications I tried failed to work. I carried a few sterile surgical instruments, and packets of surgical sponges and pads, which we prepared and sterilized in the autoclave at the hospital. I did not normally sew up any wounds or do minor surgical procedures on house calls, because I felt that it was safer to do these things in the more sterile surroundings of the office or hospital. Of course I carried the expected stethoscope and sphygmomanometer (Blood pressure cuff), reflex hammer, otoscope, tongue blades, thermometers and an opthalmoscope. Also carried were small pill dispensing boxes and envelopes, prescription pads, and occasionally pads of printed instructions for treatments. With my bag I was prepared to deal with a wide variety of medical cases.

One result of making house calls was that I soon realized that they were excellent opportunities for getting to know my patients and their families. My practice included all types of people, from the fanatically clean to the unwashed, and I quickly learned that houses had characteristic odors and smells, which reflected the people living in them. Farmhouses had definitely noticeable odors. Many of them reminded me of the smells I had experienced as a youth in my own grandmother's house. Eau de cow manure blended with a bit of hog, wet dog, wet feathers, freshly baked bread and chicken soup, etc., all blended in significant proportions, seemed to me to be representative of the people living in the house. There were also farmhouses that had no farm odors, and if there was any discernable odor at all, it was of soaps and polishes or the pine or lemon scents of cleaning materials.

The worst smelling house that I ever visited was not a farmhouse. An old lady was living in this small house with 21 cats, and when I entered the air was suffocating. The stench of cat manure was enough to cause one to gag. I had to enter that house several times before I was successful in having the county welfare people and the animal control people move her out of there. That house was so dirty that I never did set my medical bag down anywhere inside. It smelled so bad that it could not be cleaned up, but had to be destroyed. One of my friends remarked that if the house had been out in the country it would have been easiest to apply for a burning permit and burn it to the ground.

Not long after I began seeing and treating patients I realized that the great majority of people, who came to my office, did not really need medical treatment, and only a short time later I realized that most of the patients I treated at home did not really need my services either. Seldom was there a serious illness, and even more rare were the true emergencies. What most people needed was reassurance that their problem, real or perceived, would get well, or that it was not catastrophic, and they would recover or get along well in spite of it. Most importantly they wanted to be assured that, whatever the problem, they weren't going to be long suffering and were not going to die. Most people considered their doctor to be the most well educated, all-knowing oracle of information about life and medicine available, and an encouraging word from such a source usually would do much to alleviate anxiety and even lessen pain. The only thing that many patients needed was counseling. When the truth of this realization struck me I was a bit awed, and came to the conclusion that it was incumbent upon me to be completely honest with all patients regarding their medical conditions and care, because I believed that it was of prime importance to keep up my role as a medical authority, and in order to do that I couldn't be giving out false advice. I believed that in order to be believed in the future, I had to, at all times, be completely honest with my patients.

After that I always made it clear to patients and their families that I would always tell them the truth, and confide in them everything I thought about their medical problems. I regularly enlisted their help and cooperation in the treatment of their problems, because I believed that if well informed about their medical situation, they would be able to better help themselves. Furthermore, if I routinely lied to them, I would certainly not be able to remember today exactly what lie I had spoken yesterday, or the week before. I vowed that I would never allow a suspicion of prevarication to develop or grow in my relationship with my patients, because then trust between patient and doctor could not possibly be absolute.

Not only did I feel that each patient deserved to know what I thought about his/her illness, I felt that they should also be able to judge me as a physician, and in order to do that they should know as much as possible about their condition and the reasons for the treatments I prescribed. I often felt compelled to discuss these things with a patient, and particularly with the patient's family. Before long I learned that the capacity, which some persons have for absorbing any medical information at all, was severely limited. For example, I might give the family of a hospitalized stroke patient an explanation such as this:

"Brain tissue needs oxygen continuously, or it dies. Oxygen is brought to the brain in the blood, which circulates through its blood vessels. Due to the wear and tear of aging and, in Grandma's case, of high blood pressure, one of the major blood vessels in her brain has ruptured, so it can not continue to supply oxygenated blood to the part of the brain which it formerly supplied. That part of the brain has died, and included in the dead part are the nerves, which control speech and movement of the right arm and leg. Brain tissue around the dead area has been insulted by this accident, and now doesn't quite work properly. When the damage heals some of the functions of this insulted brain area may recover, but it is not likely that Grandma will ever walk again."

After having a conference with a family and having given an explanation of the illness, often more detailed than I have described here, it was very frustrating for me to hear some family member ask,

"But Doctor, what **IS** the cause of that?"

In my early practice it was not rare to have family members ask me not to tell Mother or some other sick family member that they had cancer. Never have I made such a promise, and because I always refused, I may have lost an occasional patient. The favorable side of my refusal to "hide the truth" became very obvious to me in later years, when I would be able to honestly give a patient a good prognosis, and realize that the patient gained considerable comfort and peace of mind because he/she believed me completely.

December 11, 1946 was a most memorable day for me. It began with a very early morning phone call from Detroit from my wife telling me that she was going into labor. Since this was two weeks before her due date, I told her it was most likely false labor, and to be sure it wasn't before going to the hospital. She was not happy with this diagnosis, and still to this day sometimes reminds me of it. However at the time it was quite logical to assume that she was having some false labor pains.

That morning I made rounds at the hospital, and then went to the office, where I saw a young man with classic symptoms of appendicitis. This happened to be at the time when a newly delivered mother occupied every bed in the hospital, including the beds in the labor room. So I called the administrator of Hayes-Green-Beach Hospital in Charlotte, Michigan (about 10 miles away) to ask if I could operate upon my patient there. I received a polite refusal. I could refer the patient to one of their surgeons, and could come and observe. I could also make a formal application to become a member of the medical staff there, a process that would take several weeks to be completed. So I went to Bernice and together we worked out a plan. There was only one postpartum mother in the labor room on the top floor, so we moved the other bed across the hall into the delivery room, and admitted the man there, expecting one or two of the obstetrical patients in the hospital to go home that afternoon.

Late that morning I removed my patient's inflamed appendix in the operating room at Stimson Hospital. Dr. Herman VanArk gave the open drop ether anesthesia, and seemed to be having some difficulty keeping the patient deeply anaesthetized. The surgery went well however, except that the patient squirmed a bit as I sewed up the skin. I asked Herman about it afterward and learned that he had never given an anesthetic before. This surprised me. The need was there so I urged him to learn more, which he did, and he soon became adept at administering several types of anesthesia.

Then after I left the hospital I found a number of patients waiting to see me at my office, and when I finished with them, my sister-in-law called to tell me that my wife was really in labor and had been admitted to the hospital. So early in the afternoon I set out to drive the ninety miles to Detroit, hoping to be there when she delivered. The weather was bad. Icy rain and sleet had covered the roads with an inch or more of clear ice. I thought about aborting the trip but couldn't bring myself to do it. The only safe driving speed was twenty miles per hour or less, and it took me four and one half hours to reach the hospital in Highland Park. Everywhere along the route cars had skidded off of the roads and were stuck in roadside ditches. By the time I arrived at the Highland Park General Hospital my wife had been taken to the delivery room, but I got there in time to administer some ether to her as our first-born was delivered.

The arrival of our oldest son on December 11, 1946 changed my life again. I looked upon it as the culmination of everything that had gone on before. The struggle to attain my education had been long and difficult, but I had finally accomplished it. I had the great good fortune to marry the absolutely right girl. The hardships of separation when I went into the service, and again when I went overseas into combat were difficult to bear, but we managed, and I had returned without having been killed or wounded. Finally, my medical practice had been successfully launched. Now I had a complete family of my own, and I needed to look for living quarters so that my wife and child could be with me.

Without my asking, Marian and Ralph Berg offered to let us have their master bedroom (with bath attached), while they moved in to a bedroom upstairs. Since I could find nothing even remotely suitable as living quarters for my new family, I accepted their offer, and shortly after the Christmas/New Year holiday, we moved into the Berg's downstairs master bedroom. Although far from ideal, this turned out to be a pleasant arrangement for us. The baby crib was in the bedroom. We ate with the Bergs and boarders at the big kitchen table, and I continued to carry on with my growing practice.

CHAPTER VI

THE BIG SNOW AND FLOOD

After my wife and infant son came to Eaton Rapids, things went smoothly for me. The baby was thriving. My practice was growing. I was learning a lot about the business of medicine, and was "patting myself on the back" for hiring the Professional Management team to help me run my practice. January and February passed quickly, and in March we were seeing some signs that spring was on its way.

March 23rd arrived with much rain and wind. The weather worsened early in the morning on the 24th, with the appearance of dense black clouds, lightning and thunder. A severe storm was upon us. The temperature dropped precipitously to well below freezing, and the heavy rain turned into very heavy snow, which came down so fast and so heavily that by early evening the surrounding country roads became snowed in, and traffic could not pass. By evening even the State Highway, M-50, was snowbound.

That was when the phone rang. There was a woman in labor in a farmhouse near Narrow Lake, which was some eight or nine miles from downtown. The Webster Lumber & Coal Yard was contributing a Caterpillar tractor, with a small trailer attached, and a driver to take me out to her. Would I please ride out there in the trailer to help the woman?

I promptly agreed to go, but went first to the hospital for some supplies. Bernice had been forewarned that I was coming, and had prepared a large picnic basket with an obstetric pack containing sterile drapes and instruments, separately wrapped obstetrical forceps, and vials of anesthetic solution to be used if needed to repair any lacerations or an episiotomy incision. Warmly dressed, carrying my medical bag in one hand and the picnic basket of medical supplies on the other arm, I met the tractor and its driver in the center of town. I had never met the driver before. He was introduced to me only as Willard.

With Willard in the driver's seat of the tractor, I climbed into the four foot by eight-foot trailer box, and knelt down near the front of it. Soon we were off down Main Street, going south, out of town. There were onlookers present to see us off, but we quickly left them behind. It was still snowing hard, and blowing winds were causing huge snowdrifts to form. After we had gone about two miles south on the highway, with the steel-treaded tractor ever seeming to climb up upon the snow and at the same time crush it down, our route took us East on a country road. After only a short distance in the new direction, we ran into serious trouble. The snow was so deep that in order to go forward the tractor had to continually climb up in the snowdrifts. With the tractor treads continually climbing upward at a thirty to forty-five degree angle with the road surface, we seemed to be constantly climbing uphill. This resulted in the trailer digging into the fallen snow so deeply that the tractor could no longer pull it. What to do?

We unhitched the trailer, and Willard and I both got up on the tractor, each of us having one half of the metal bucket seat to sit on. Willard was on the left, and driving the tractor. I was on the right, with the picnic basket still on my arm, clutching my medical bag, and bracing my feet and legs to keep from falling off. Now the tractor could go forward. With its nose pointing upward and its rear seemingly below the surface of the snow, it seemed that the faster we went the easier it became, much like a speedboat traveling at high speed and planing across the surface of a lake. In places along the route the snow must have been fifteen or more feet deep, as judged by the amount of the hedgerow treetops I saw protruding above its surface. Sitting on the rim of that bucket seat wasn't very comfortable, so we were lucky that the tractor could make good speed, and we were able to reach our destination earlier than we had expected.

We drove into the farmyard and up to the door of the house. I jumped off of the tractor still clutching my bag and the picnic basket, to be met at the door by anxious family members, and I was immediately directed in to see the patient. This was her first baby, and so far the length of the labor had been about average. I observed immediately that the baby's head was crowning, i.e. it had already descended so far down the birth canal that it was spreading the exterior tissues apart. A substantial area of the baby's scalp was showing.

There was no time to apply the sterile obstetrical drapes, or to even scrub my hands and apply sterile gloves, because I got my first view of the situation while the patient was having a labor contraction and had a very strong, unstoppable urge to push the baby out. Before I had time to do anything I saw the patient's stretched out perineum split wide open. The baby came out in a rush, cried almost immediately, and appeared to be in excellent condition. We waited then for the placenta (afterbirth) to separate, and when the signs of separation appeared I was able to express it with what we called the Crede maneuver. Then I gave the mother an ampoule of ergotrate, hypodermically, to cause the uterus to contract and stay contracted, and thus minimize postpartum bleeding.

Now the only thing left to do was to repair the fairly extensive laceration of the perineum. It was what we called a second-degree tear, i.e.

it tore the surface tissues and the muscle below, but did not tear the rectum or any of the rectal muscles.

No problem!! I opened the picnic basket which Bernice had so carefully prepared, and at about that time was told that a phone call had come reporting that there was another young woman in labor in a farmhouse about two miles away. Willard and I agreed that we would go there as soon as I was finished here. I looked in the basket, and picked out a vial of local anesthetic, some topical antiseptic, a packet of sterile rubber gloves, a sterile obstetric repair kit containing hemostats, needle holders and some other surgical instruments. There were sterile surgical needles, BUT WHERE WERE THE SUTURES, the stitching materials needed to sew up the wound??? Bernice had forgotten to include them in the basket!

Now I had to think. What to do? If I didn't repair the tear, the perineum would take much longer to heal up, but there shouldn't be any other problems. After all, failure to repair perineal tears had probably occurred thousands of times in past history, and most of those women had survived. On the other hand there were a lot of older women with cystocoeles, rectocoeles, and prolapsed uteri, which made them miserable, and I did not want anything like that to happen to this new mother. Finally I asked if there was any black silk thread in the house. Yes there was. I went with one of the women to a sewing machine, and picked out a spool of heavy black silk thread. I peeled off about a dozen one foot lengths, and sterilized them as best I could by boiling them for a time in clean water in a clean pot on the cook-stove. Then I scrubbed my hands, applied sterile gloves, washed the laceration and the perineum several times with antiseptic, and injected the area with local anesthetic solution. I did, however, not do this repair in the usual fashion. Instead I placed interrupted stitches of that black silk in what is usually described as "figure of eight" stitches. The deep loop of the "eight" encircled all of the tissues except the skin and some of the fat under the skin, and brought the two sides together again in approximately normal position. Then instead of tying them I crossed the threads and brought them out through the skin on the opposite sides to complete the figure eight. When they were tied, the deep tissues, including the muscles, were held in approximation by the deep loop of the "eight" and the skin was held closed by the superficial loop. The advantage of stitches like this was that no suture material had to remain permanently in the wound, and if any sign of abnormal inflammation or infection occurred in any of them, the offending one or two or three stitches could be prematurely removed without disrupting the wound. I felt that this was important, because I could not be sure that just boiling that black silk thread really made it surgically sterile.

Before we left to go to the next case, I left some ergotrate tablets for the new mother to take to keep the uterus contracted, some instructions on breast feeding and perineal care, on how to prepare an infant formula with evaporated milk and Karo Syrup, and a prescription for vitamins for the baby. The mother was to report any significant fever or unusual increase in perineal pain, and was to come in to the office in one week to have the stitches removed. When she arrived at my office a week later, the perineum was healing beautifully, and I was able to remove all of those black silk stitches.

As soon as I was able to leave this patient we were off to the next case. As I mounted that half tractor seat once again, I remembered that I had not used the obstetrical drapes in the basket and I was glad, because it was quite likely that I would want to use them for the next delivery. It was still snowing but no longer so very windy. We made good time on the tractor, and soon arrived at the next farmhouse. As I was ushered in I observed that this house was more poorly and sparsely furnished than the first one had been. There was a wood cooking range in the kitchen, but the fire had gone out. There was a small pot-bellied stove in the dining room, which seemed to be burning briskly, but in spite of that the room seemed cold. Behind a closed door to a bedroom, which opened off of the dining room, was the patient in labor.

The room was dark as I entered, except for a small amount of light coming in from the dining room. A hodge-podge tangle of blankets, quilts, sheets, towels and probably other items of cloth was piled high on the large double bed in a heap that covered most of the mattress. I saw no sign of anyone in labor, but quickly spotted a column of steam rising from this heap through a hole in the pile near the head of the bed. It was the patient's breath. It was so cold in the room that the laboring mother's breath was visible.

These were impossible conditions under which to deliver a baby, so I asked immediately for a cot with a mattress to be put into the dining room in front of the stove. Fortunately there were such items somewhere in the house. With the mattress protected with multiple layers of newspaper, we moved the patient out into the dining room and onto the cot, and supplied her with some decent blankets. I told the family members to start a fire in the kitchen stove and stay in there. Some of the boys (young men) went outside to saw up some old telephone poles and split the wood for the stove. It was now after midnight, the beginning of a new day, March 25th.

This was also a first baby for this young woman. After examining her I estimated that she was about three quarters of the way through labor. The baby's position in the uterus and birth canal was satisfactory, the cervix had already dilated to about 7 centimeters, and the baby's heartbeat sounded fine. I explained the situation to Willard, my tractor driver, and told him that I would have to stay until the baby was born. He decided not to wait, and left on the tractor immediately to go back to town. I had known Willard only a few hours, and didn't know his last name. Much later I learned that his full name was Willard Desgrange. He worked for the Webster family on their farmland and in the lumber and coal yard. He lived some distance from town, and that is probably why our paths did not cross again.

Labor continued with vigorous, regular contractions every two to three minutes. I stayed with my patient and gave her an injection to take the edge off of the labor pains. I rechecked my picnic basket. When the time came I would use the sterile obstetrical drapes. But now my chief concern was that an episiotomy might be needed, or that the patient might sustain a perineal tear, which would require a repair procedure. I still had sterile syringes and local anesthetic available for use, but if repairs were needed it would be necessary to somehow re-sterilize the instruments and some thread. Silk was considered to be best but I knew that if none was available, I could safely use cotton.

The patient was an absolute jewel. I knew that she was having pain and that she was frightened, but I coached her, and she did everything I told her to do, including NOT BEARING DOWN OR PUSHING WHEN THE PERINEUM WAS BEING STRETCHED TO ITS LIMIT BY THE BABY'S HEAD DURING A CONTRACTION. After the head started to crown (show outside) I applied the sterile drapes, donned the rubber gloves, and concentrated upon trying to get the baby's head born without allowing any lacerations to occur. Some twelve to fifteen contractions were needed to stretch the perineum completely, and during them I cautioned the patient not to push hard. Sometimes I held the head back a bit. Then with the last contraction the baby's head came through easily, and there were no lacerations.

After the umbilical cord had been cut and tied, and the placenta delivered, I gave the mother the usual injection of ergotrate to keep the uterus contracted, and left several ergotrate tablets in a packet on the table for her later use. Then with mother lying quietly in her cot bed by the stove in the dining room, with the baby lying quietly beside her, I looked at my watch. It was just past 5:00 AM. I went into the bedroom where I had first found the laboring mother, crawled into the bed fully clothed, covered up with the tangle on it, and slept soundly for about five hours.

When I awoke it was broad daylight. The storm had stopped, and patches of sunshine were showing. With not much wind outside, the house seemed warmer. My patient appeared to be recovering nicely. I was invited to some breakfast in the kitchen and had some coffee and ate some cereal. We were still snowed in, but I declined the offer to stay the day, and carrying my doctor bag and my picnic basket I started out to walk back to town. The snow was about waist deep most of the way, and the going was very slow, but I was in good physical condition and made good progress. People in the farmhouses along the way knew what I what doing, and seemed to be expecting me. Wherever I came abreast a farmyard someone would be out to greet me and ask me in for food and coffee. I accepted only a few of these invitations, but there were enough of them that people in town could keep accurate track of my progress, because the telephones were working.

By the time I reached Highway M-50 it was well after dark, and by then the highway department snowplows had managed to clear the road out that far from town. Wayne Gibson, the local Ford dealer, met me there in his car, and brought me home. He agreed that this had been the worst snowstorm that he had ever seen, and told me that Dr. Goff had also gone out into the storm to take care of a patient, and he had ridden a horse!

When I got back to the Webster House that evening, I thought that the ordeal of the late season storm was over, but I was wrong. It was cold in the house, and everyone was dressed as if they were outdoors. All of them complained that they had headaches. The electric power had failed during the storm, and since it was an entirely electric house, everything but the city water and sewer was out of operation. Our baby son seemed to do well with extra blankets and bottle feedings warmed on the open oven door over some burning candles. My wife cheerfully reported that two candles warmed the bottle almost twice as fast as one. With no electricity we could not cook, and we had no light except for candles. The house was cold because it had a coal furnace, which was fed by a coal stoker, and without electricity the stoker did not run.

Mrs. Berg had fussed with the furnace, trying to keep a coal fire burning in it while the stoker was not working, and when I went down into the basement to check on it there were indeed a few glowing coals in the middle of the firepot. It seemed to me that without the stoker running not enough air could enter the firepot to sustain the burning very well. There was also a smoke smell in the basement, which I had not detected upstairs. So I stepped around behind the furnace and found the smoke pipe, which led to the brick chimney. It was about eight feet long and contained a damper, which when opened would allow basement air to be sucked up the chimney, when necessary, to slow the draft leaving the firepot. I lifted the damper flap and with the aid of a flashlight found that this smoke pipe, which was about ten inches in diameter, was so badly clogged with thick, black soot, that its actual working diameter inside must have been less than two inches.

At that point a light dawned in my mind. All of the adults upstairs complained of headache and this probably meant CARBON MONOXIDE POISONING!!!!!!! I rushed upstairs, and in spite of the cold we opened doors and windows wide, to blow out whatever carbon monoxide might be there. I went back down in the cellar and checked the fire in the furnace. What little was left appeared to be going out, so I left it alone, but pulled the switches so that the stoker system would not start up again when the electric power came back on. When I went back down a short time later, the fire had indeed gone out.

After the whole house was thoroughly aired out, we closed the doors and windows, and spent the rest of the night in the cold house. There were plenty of blankets available, so it wasn't uncomfortable to be in bed. The power came back on before morning, and Mrs. Berg reported the furnace problem to the Webster Coal & Lumber business, which had not only installed the stoker but also supplied the coal. That afternoon while the house was still quite cold, Mary VanAuker appeared at our door with a big pot of hot, delicious, homemade vegetable soup, which was much appreciated. It tasted exceptionally good, and warmed us all inside! The furnace was quickly repaired, and before the end of the day was safely in service again, but it took another twenty-four hours for that big house to feel comfortably warm inside. I thought then that we were finished with that storm and the troubles that came with it. But once again I was wrong!

About one week after that very heavy snowfall we suffered another heavy snowstorm during one evening and overnight. Then the weather warmed up considerably, and seemed to accelerate the snowmelt. Since we were already in the month of April, temperatures remained above freezing most of the time. By looking through the back windows of the Webster House we could see the Grand River flowing past the yard, and we could also see most of the island in the river. We first noticed that the water had risen to cover the island's edges and portions of the lawn. After some hours we found the entire lawn submerged. Then the water gradually rose to cover the cannon mounts, and finally rose to cover the cannons completely. Only the upper few feet of the gazebo and the big trees remained visible above water. By that time the middle block of Main Street, where my office was located, was also under water. The sidewalk in front of my office was submerged under half of a foot of water, and when I checked, I found that the water in my basement had risen to within about three inches of the surface of my office floor. The report came to us that some boys were catching bullheads out of the basement at the bank, which was located at the North end of the same city block in which my office was located. All of that part of Main Street that was on the downtown "island" had standing water on it. The streets to the North and to the South had higher elevations, and were not flooded, so there was no problem getting to the hospital, but I did not open my office for several days. Water Street, which runs along the West side of the river, appeared to have been aptly named, because much of the first mile or two out from downtown was also under water.

Once the crest of the flood had passed the waters receded steadily. Main Street was not inundated for very long, but it took a long time for the water in my office basement to disappear. Eventually it did, and the basement also dried out well. Descriptions of the snowstorm and flood circulated about town for a number of years afterward, but up to the present time Main Street has never been flooded again.

After the waters had receded and I could work in my office again, I spent most of my time working. I continued to accept a lot of house calls because I was concerned about whether or not my practice would be successful, and this soon entailed a considerable amount of night work. I soon became chronically tired, but I didn't mind that, because my practice was growing. It was especially gratifying to see my list of obstetrical patients grow.

When I started my practice there was no formal emergency room or emergency service available in Eaton Rapids. Serious cases of illness or injury were taken by ambulance to the hospital, where they could have their regular doctor or their doctor of choice called in to attend them. Most times the doctor was called first, and the decision to go by ambulance to the hospital was made during a phone conversation ahead of time. Soon by mutual agreement, Dr. Bert VanArk, Dr Herman VanArk and I worked out a system for covering each other's practices, when necessary. This gave each of us some nighttime rest.

Edmere and I continued to live with our first-born in the Webster House, but I had Mr. Heminger continue to look for housing for us that we could afford. At that time my father was also in the real estate sales business in Detroit, and he visited us in Eaton Rapids often. On every visit he consulted with Mr. Heminger to see if any type of housing had become available, and my father and Roy Heminger became well acquainted. The two real estate salesmen had much in common. Roy kept calling my Dad "Mister Minkey," and my Dad called Roy "Mister Hemingway."

Then one day in the late Spring Dad met me in the hospital with the news that a house had been found for us. All I would need was enough money for a required down payment. Fortunately there were just enough dollars in the bank to cover it. In the months that I had been in practice we had lived very frugally, and I had saved as much money as possible for this very purpose. Soon Edmere and I were the owners of an old house with a substantial mortgage at 208 Dutton Street. We moved in as soon as we could, and made it our home.

The house stood on a nice big lot on the corner of River and Dutton Streets. There were several mature Northern Spy apple trees, and some maple and ash trees on the property, and it had a two-car garage that opened upon its own driveway on River Street. We were told that the house had been built at about the time of the Civil War, and it was obvious that the single story kitchen and dining room was a later addition. The house had what was called a Michigan cellar, a shallow basement with sloping dirt walls. In it was a furnace with a coal stoker, and there was a stairway to the outside covered by a double, hatch-like door which was weatherproof to keep the rain out. Floors in the main part of the house sagged a bit, and when we engaged a carpenter to cut a door from the living room into the dining room, he found that the wall, which had once been an outside wall of the house, was built of solid hard maple, four inches thick. There were two layers of rough-sawn, maple boards, each two inches thick. In one layer the boards were horizontal and in the other they were vertical. This wall was difficult to cut through, and when finished we found that the living room floor was about four inches lower than the dining room floor. We had it finished off to include a stair step there. Later we had a larger window cut into the kitchen, and had similar difficulty with the wall there.

In spite of a dearth of furnishings, we settled into our new home quickly. We brought in some of the waiting room chairs that had been in the Gunnell Barber shop. Kitchen stove, refrigerator, automatic washing machine and a pine bedroom set were bought very inexpensively from the man for whom I had worked when I was in high school, and we transported them ourselves from Detroit. They had been items for sale in his business that had not moved for a long time, and I suspect that he let me have them for even less than their original wholesale price.

We still had our 1941 Studebaker Champion automobile that we had been fortunate enough to purchase soon after I came home from overseas, which was about a year before I was separated from the service. I used it in my practice, and depended so much on it that Edmere did not have much time with it. She used it for short periods of time only, and often walked downtown to the stores. Milk was delivered to our door from Williams Dairy, usually by Max Williams himself with his horse and wagon.

CHAPTER VII

THE SWITCH TO GROUP PRACTICE

By mid-summer of my first year in practice everything seemed to be going well. I was working long hours, and my practice was growing. Patients were returning after an initial consultation, and I had already seen some of them several times. The arrangement I had with the VanArks for mutual call coverage was also working well, and it gave me a little time off for rest. I no longer felt as if I was on the verge of exhaustion. Our arrangement also resulted in the three of us going together in one car to the monthly county medical society meetings in Charlotte. As we gained knowledge about each other and the way we practiced medicine, a mutual respect developed. We were "good" doctors, with good medical educations, who handled patients sympathetically and treated them conservatively.

This was the situation when, early in the fall, Dr. Bert VanArk reported that Bernice Bowman had approached him with a proposition. She and Mrs. Stimson no longer wanted to own the hospital and wanted to sell it. They asked $25,000 for the whole thing,-------- land, building, furniture, fixtures, all of the medical supplies and equipment. Further, the ladies proposed a sales contract in which there would be no interest charged on the outstanding balance. In addition, Bernice would continue to work for us as the hospital administrator. All we would need to do was make monthly payments, all of which would be applied to reduce the principal owed.

Dr. Bert, Dr. Herman and I discussed the offer, and realized that the conditions of such a contract were most favorable to us. We decided to form a practice partnership, and have the partnership buy the hospital under those terms. We could turn the main floor of the hospital building into satisfactory office space with a minimum of remodeling. We would give up our offices downtown, practice from within the hospital itself, and by doing so we would be saving the expense of maintaining our separate downtown offices. Little did we realize the consequences of this arrangement. Having the doctors' offices in the hospital lobby, a place that never closes, would make it very difficult for us to go home in time for dinner in the evenings, because patients would continue to come in after hours for service.

There was a delay while written partnership agreements and documents for the sale were prepared, but the remodeling started very soon. The far end of the lobby was walled off, making a large room, which became my examining room and also doubled as an emergency room. The areas on both sides of the corridor to the elevator were divided into more examining rooms as was the space which had formerly been Dr. Stimson's office, and a part of it was used as our business office. We decided to name the new partnership the Stimson Medical Group, and had stationery and prescription pads prepared with the new name. When the Christmas holidays arrived preparations for our move into the hospital were progressing well.

My wife and I wanted to visit our respective families in Detroit on Christmas Eve and Christmas Day, and Dr. Herman VanArk wanted to visit family during the same time. Dr. Bert VanArk agreed to cover for us while we were gone. When we returned the news was all over town that Dr. Sidney Goff had committed suicide in his office by slashing his wrists. Dr. Bert was the one who had to go in and pronounce him dead, and I could see in his demeanor that it had been a most difficult duty. Indeed it shocked and saddened us all.

Some time in about the middle of January, 1948, after all business arrangements had been completed and furnishings and equipment had been moved from our downtown offices, we opened our offices in the hospital, and began practicing there as the Stimson Medical Group. Ours was one of the first medical group practices in Michigan, and after we had operated only a short time, it became apparent that this type of practice offered advantages for both doctor and patient. Pooling our resources and sharing employees produced significant financial savings. Because our offices were now in the hospital less travel time was necessary. During office hours, we (doctors) could and did often call upon each other for an opinion on what we considered to be a difficult case while the patient was still in the office. This in effect gave the patient a quick second opinion, and bolstered everyone's faith in the treatment prescribed. At that time, and never in all of the years that I practiced in the group, did we ever charge the patient anything for the second opinion.

Another advantage was that surgery, labor and delivery rooms were almost instantly available upstairs, as were hospital beds for admitting patients, so no time was wasted in driving back and forth. Indeed, when we had a mother-to-be in labor upstairs in the hospital, we could continue our office practice until she was ready, and then run upstairs to deliver the baby. We could often be back downstairs to continue office hours in twenty minutes or so.

We established our practice pharmacy in the hospital laboratory room on the main floor, and kept our injectable medicines and the medicines we dispensed there. Upstairs on the main patient floor was another pharmacy stocked with medicines for hospital inpatients. We had no laboratory technicians. The office assistants did the most simple laboratory tests needed for our office practices, such as testing urine for albumin and sugar, and the hospital floor nurses did the same for the hospital inpatients. The doctors did whatever other tests they required and were able to do, and oversaw the mailing of specimens for more complicated testing in an out of town laboratory.

The laboratory equipment that we had was quite fundamental. My microscope was used in the lab to examine urine sediment, blood and bacterial smears, and to do blood counts using dilution pipettes and a counting chamber. We had stains for blood smears, and in addition did some gram stains to help identify bacteria. Occasionally we used acid-fast stains to try to detect tubercle bacilli. We had a centrifuge with appropriate centrifuge tubes for examining urine sediment and determining hematocrit levels. There were several extra hemoglobinometers available, and we used them often. We frequently checked the hemoglobin levels of our obstetrical patients while they were undergoing prenatal care to be sure that none would be anemic at the time of delivery. In those days we had no great interest in exact identification of bacteria so did not do bacterial cultures very often. When identification was crucial we sent the specimens to the Michigan State Laboratory, or occasionally to another outside laboratory to be processed and read.

Blood transfusions were not possible for us. Although it was possible for us to do the blood typing and cross matching ourselves, we felt that because we would not be doing these things very often, there would be too much room for error in the test results. In emergencies, when the necessity for transfusion seemed imminent, we could only administer intravenous salt solutions or freeze dried plasma, and transfer the patient as an emergency to a Lansing hospital as quickly as possible.

Serology tests for syphilis, required by law, were done at the State Laboratory. We sent the blood samples for all of our obstetrical patients and many of our hospital inpatients there. Our tissue specimens were examined by the Pathology Department at the University of Michigan. We mailed them there, and in less than a week received a detailed report, usually including a definite pathological diagnosis made by an expert in the field.

Our business office was headed by Mrs. Mary Jordan, who had been the bookkeeper in the VanArk office before the move. She and Bernice collaborated and did all of the accounting, billing, payroll preparation, and bill paying for both the hospital and the medical group. There were a few years then when I did not have Professional Management oversee my business, but later, after the medical group had grown, I convinced my partners to hire Professional Management again.

The remaining larger portion of what had been hospital lobby now doubled as our office waiting room. An ordinary desk with a telephone was placed at the far end from the main entrance, and presiding over it was our receptionist, who was also charged with taking telephone calls, delivering messages, and handling requests for office appointments. In my opinion this was the worst job in the clinic, and if not properly done it could make everyone, including the jobholder, miserable. We hired a number of women in succession into that position. Some didn't like it, and didn't last long in the job. Some did seem to like it and got along quite well, but the one who lives in my memory as being the best is Vonda Thompson, who held the position for a long time. Her parents were patients of mine before she worked for us, and they remained favorite patients until I retired from practice. Vonda could make decisions and take charge of whatever situation she faced, and she could do it without seeming to seriously offend anyone.

CHAPTER VIII

EARLY CHANGES IN MEDICAL PRACTICE

In January 1948 when Dr. Bert VanArk, Dr. Herman VanArk and I merged our practices together, named ourselves the Stimson Medical Group, and moved our offices from downtown to the main floor of the hospital, we also made some changes in the way we practiced. First, we changed the way medical records were made and kept, to a system in which there was only one clinical record for each patient. We used the full-page sized forms that Professional Management had recommended. Each patient record was kept in a standard, letter-sized file folder, and each patient visit was recorded in it by the doctor who had seen the patient. Records of subsequent visits, no matter which doctor may have been consulted, were added to this same record. Thus a patient's clinical record might contain entries made by one or all of the group's doctors. In later years, as the size of the medical group grew, there could be as many as eleven doctors who had made entries into a patient's single clinical record.

Another change which was unplanned, but which seemed to have happened more or less spontaneously as a result of our practicing in the same office, was the immediate availability of a second, although informal, medical opinion. Whenever doctor or patient had doubts about a diagnosis or treatment, it was a simple process to have one of the other physicians step into the room, review the case, render his opinion, and perhaps influence the choice of treatment. These second opinion consultations were always informal. The consulting physician did not write into the patient record, but the primary physician often made note of his opinion when he recorded the information regarding that specific clinical visit. These second opinion consultations were always free, and no charge for them was made to the patient.

During the following several years changes in actual medical practice occurred. One of the first was to get the newly delivered mothers up and out of bed within hours of their delivery. We all felt that this was important in order to keep their blood circulation robust and healthy, and prevent clot formation (thrombosis), especially in the deep leg veins. The new mothers seemed to show no resistance to this practice, but there was definitely opposition to it from mother-in-laws and grandmothers, who felt that ten days of bed rest after childbirth was absolutely necessary for healing to take place. This belief was prevalent among the women of the older generations, and after I had practiced in Eaton Rapids for a time, I believed that I knew why they felt this way.

Before World War II childbirth was usually attended by persons, including doctors, with varying degrees of knowledge and skill. Birth canal injuries often went unrecognized, were more or less ignored or were, by modern standards, inadequately repaired. Post partum hemorrhage was a serious and feared complication. Unless the new mother had a disorder in which her blood would not clot, fatal hemorrhage from a normal post partum uterus was practically impossible. Excessive post-partum bleeding was often due to small pieces of placenta breaking off and remaining behind in the uterus after the placenta had been delivered. Sometimes the fragments of placenta left behind had to be removed, but often these small pieces would later be spontaneously expelled from the uterus, and from then on the amount of bloody vaginal discharge would remain normal. Bleeding from tears in the lower vagina and perineum were not likely to ever be fatal. Lacerations of the upper vagina, the cervix, and the uterus itself are easy to overlook, and because they are hidden, could be the cause of continued bleeding which, unless stopped, could result in bleeding to death. Bleeding of this type is aggravated by any movements, which cause disturbance of the torn tissues. Blood clots, which have formed to stem the bleeding, are disturbed, and fall away from the bleeding points. The result is repeated restarting or continuation of the bleeding. In spite of this danger, some, perhaps many, of these cases survived, if they were kept quietly in bed for a prolonged period of time, i.e. long enough for the clots to solidify and permanently shut down the blood loss.

All damages suffered by the birth canal during childbirth, when healed, result in structural changes in it. The more severe the injuries are, the more severe are the structural and functional changes that result, and in many cases they cause dysfunction and disability.

After I had examined a number of older women in the area, and listened to their complaints, it appeared to me that in the past there had been a high incidence of obstetrical injuries with resulting malfunctions and deformities in the local population. Cystocoele (bulging of the bladder), rectocoele (bulging of the rectum), and often both together were a relatively common problem. Cystocoele often caused incontinence of urine, and rectocoele contributed to constipation. When these bulges became large enough to protrude from the vagina, vaginal mucous membrane would be exposed outside of the vagina when the woman stood up. This caused problems with sanitation, as well as gave the woman the feeling that her "bottom" was falling out. Then there was a condition known as uterine prolapse (dropped uterus), which occurred in several degrees. It was not rare in those times. I had several older patients in whom the uterine ligaments had been so stretched and the vaginal walls and uterine support structures had become so attenuated that the uterus dropped completely out through the vagina and remained there as long as the patient remained standing. In two of my patients the condition had existed so long that the vaginal mucous membrane, now exposed in almost its entirety, had dried up and changed to something that resembled the outside skin of the body. At the far end of this protuberance was the uterine cervix, and the whole thing bore an uncanny resemblance to an elephant's trunk. Another condition, which looked similar to a rectocoele, was what was called an enterocoele, which is actually an abdominal hernia, which protrudes down out of the abdominal cavity through an enlarged gap just behind the uterus and presents itself coming out of the vagina. Fortunately enterocoeles were not common, because these hernias are not only difficult to recognize but are difficult to repair. Although many surgical operations had been proposed and were being done to correct birth canal deformities, none were perfect, and few were without their own problems. Before World War II the more difficult and serious deformities could not be surgically fixed outside of a University Medical Center or other large, similarly skilled institutions.

A common way to treat prolapse and vaginal protrusions in the past was the use of pessaries, which are apparatuses placed into the vagina to hold the uterus and its attached tissues up inside. I saw many of them, but did not often prescribe one myself, preferring to offer some type of surgical repair instead. Fat and thin doughnut shapes, bell shapes and toadstool shapes, designed so that the stem remained in the lower vagina and kept the cap pointed in the right direction, were common. Two or three times in my career I saw an old lady for the first time who had had a pessary inserted years before, and it had remained inside for many years. To these poor women a malodorus vaginal discharge was a normal condition of life.

Certainly there were causes for these birth canal problems. Some were obvious and some not so obvious. In my opinion the cause most often responsible for them was the advice that was almost universally given to the laboring mothers-to-be by attendants (family members, nurses, midwives, and yes, even doctors), to bear down. "Push! Push haaaaard!!! Hold your breath and puuuuuush!!!!"

The consequence of following such instruction before the uterine contractions had fully dilated the cervix, would be to force the baby's head, still encased in the partially dilated cervix, down into the pelvis, without any possibility of delivering it. Such bearing down forces the incompletely dilated cervix down into the pelvis, tends to bruise it and cause it to swell, overstretches the uterine support structures, and actually interferes with cervical dilation. Furthermore, all of these "battered" tissues become more prone to injury during the delivery, especially if it is a difficult one or forceps are used. I have never urged a laboring woman to push or bear down under these circumstances, and I have more than once been called to see one who has been laboring and bearing down prematurely. Usually, if I am able to convince her to stop pushing for eight or ten normal contractions, the cervical dilation will complete itself and delivery will become relatively easy. In many cases women have volunteered information to me after their delivery,

"I didn't need to be told to push. When the time came I couldn't stop pushing."

This always served to reinforce my opinion that it is not necessary to urge a laboring mother-to-be to PUUUUUUUUSH!!!!

In difficult labors and deliveries we had been taught how to apply and use obstetrical forceps of various types to assist in the birth, or sometimes to actually extract the baby's head. Forceps were sometimes blamed for birth canal injuries, and, indeed, they could cause all manner of damage if carelessly used. I suspected that forceps use was a prime cause of laceration of the upper vagina and uterine cervix, which were injuries often unsuspected and overlooked. Even if overlooked, such injuries would usually heal, aided by the rich blood supply to the tissues in the female pelvis. The result, however, would be a deformed birth canal.

Another major cause for birth canal deformities was failure to properly repair tears (lacerations). I suspected that a birth injury occurring on the inside of the birth canal often went unrecognized, and no attempt at repair was made. Failure to properly repair an episiotomy wound (an incision in the perineum purposely made to enlarge the vaginal opening) also had its consequences. A good repair involved putting the cut or torn tissues back together with careful approximation of each tissue layer to its counterpart on the opposite side of the incision. This is especially true in what we call second-degree tears, in which muscle in the perineum is torn, and it is imperative in third degree tears in which rectal wall and/or rectal sphincter muscle is torn. In many cases such repairs are complicated by the fact that the tissues of opposing sides will be asymmetrically stretched, often resulting in tremendous distortions. It seemed to be common practice in the past to just approximate the two sides of an episiotomy with large stitches so that the gross appearance of the repair appeared to be normal, but without considering the relative positions of component structures underneath the skin. Often the layers did line up well in spite of big stitches, and the repair turned out to be adequate with a good final result. However, it was quite common in middle aged and older women to see a condition which we called "relaxed perineum", which I believe is the result of inadequately bringing together an episiotomy or a tear into that area of the birth canal. An enlarged vaginal opening through which a bit of bulging rectum can usually be seen is the usual end result.

Infection in the wounds that resulted from childbirth was another problem, which often resulted in some type of birth canal deformity. We were not a great many years past the discovery that post partum infection, often called puerpueral sepsis, was caused by germs carried into the vagina and uterus from one patient to another on the hands of obstetricians. Once this concept was firmly established, strict sterile technique as practiced in the hospital surgical suites was practiced in obstetrical deliveries, and post partum infections decreased rapidly in number. Another thing that contributed considerably to this decrease was the strict observance of avoiding entering the vagina during labor with hand or instrument in order to avoid getting outside bacteria into the birth canal. When I was trained it was a serious breach of practice to do a vaginal examination of a woman in labor without first doing a surgical preparation of the birth canal and external genitalia with antiseptic solutions, and then use sterile gloves and drapes. I was taught to determine the amount of cervical dilatation during labor by doing rectal examinations, in which a finger inserted into the laboring woman's rectum was used to feel and delineate the rim of the cervix. I am sure that some practitioners did not get the hang of it very well. This is not an easy examination to do, because the thinned out cervix often had to be felt through the several distinct layers of anterior rectal wall and posterior vaginal wall. It is easy to miss feeling the lip of a cervix that is eighty to ninety percent dilated, and think that the cervix is completely dilated. The patient is then rushed into the delivery room. A surgical prep is done, and sterile drapes applied. Now the patient is ready for delivery, only to have the obstetrician discover that the cervix has not yet completely dilated. Under these circumstances, particularly during my internship, I have heard attending physicians urge their patients to PUSH.

With the passage of years it has now become normal for obstetricians to do vaginal examinations during labor using minimum sterile precautions. I realize that this practice allows for the much more accurate determination of the progress of the labor, and is in the long run better for the patient and the baby, but I still feel uncomfortable about the possibility of transmitting infection during labor, and feel that it is the advent of multiple antibiotics that has given the obstetricians license to do vaginal examinations so freely during labor.

The human body has powerful recuperative ability and is able to heal even large wounds. I believe that in the years before I began medical practice, invisible, unrecognized, and un-repaired birth canal damage occurred quite often, and healed, resulting in the birth canal disfigurements that I have discussed. These are, I repeat, relaxed perineum, cystocoele, rectocoele, enterocoele, various degrees of uterine prolapse, and combinations of several of these things occurring together. I am happy to report that after the younger physicians were released from their military service in World War II, obstetrical practice improved noticeably, and these unfortunate after effects of childbirth occurred less and less often. When they did, they were generally less severe.

Anesthesia for childbirth also took a big step forward in those early years. Not long after I started practice my wife and I visited some friends we had made while I was in the Army. He was then a resident physician in Obstetrics and Gynecology at Flower Fifth Avenue Hospital in New York, and I was able to spend several days sharing his residency there with him. I learned the techniques known as saddle block anesthesia using "heavy" nupercaine, which was great for eliminating much labor pain without stopping the labor, and pudendal block with procaine, which worked excellently in the cases where careful repair of the posterior vaginal wall and perineum were needed. It turned out to be ideal for the repair of most episiotomies. When we returned from New York, I introduced these practices to my local colleagues, and we were using saddle block anesthesia for deliveries in Eaton Rapids before it became routine anywhere else in the area.

Another practice that we followed, which was not common at the time, was to allow the father of the baby about to be born into the delivery room to observe the birth of his child. In those times this was a huge taboo everywhere else, and to the best of my knowledge we were doing it in Eaton Rapids long before it became common practice in Michigan. I am not sure that we started the practice, but I invited the father into the delivery room at my first delivery, and every one after that. Some simple precautions were taken. The father washed his hands thoroughly, was given a cap, mask and gown to wear, and was told not to touch anything, no matter what was going on. Whenever a father declined to attend, I invited a grandmother or an aunt in to observe the delivery and offer reassurance and encouragement to the mother. Occasionally a father would be overcome by his wife's difficulties, or perhaps by the sight of blood. Usually he turned pale, excused himself and left the room. I do not remember that any father ever fainted, and only once in my whole career did I ask an expectant father to leave the delivery room. He didn't object to leaving, and later several of my friends, who had seen him, told me that he had returned to the tavern from whence he had come to observe the birth.

We had been in practice for several years when St. Lawrence Hospital in Lansing renovated its obstetrical suite, and offered us an obstetrical delivery table that they were replacing. We accepted instantly. I believe we may have paid them a token price for it, and I'm sure that we paid the cost of having it moved. It would make the delivery processes, such as maintaining a sterile field, and positioning the patient to good advantage, much easier, and it would be much more comfortable for the mother than was possible with the two wooden boxes we were using.

There was one problem however. The new table with its gadgets and extensions was too large and bulky to fit comfortably into our narrow delivery room. Moving the delivery room across the hall into what had been the labor room, and moving the labor room, which needed only two beds, into the old delivery room, easily solved this problem, and we were in business.

There is a baby that I delivered in the old delivery room before the move, that I would like to mention, because he is an example of the tenacity of human life. It was not the first delivery for this mother. She was quite well along in the labor, but when I examined her, I found to my surprise that, since her last prenatal examination in the office, the baby had turned into a breech presentation. Sometimes this circumstance is a subtle warning that something is not right in the uterus. It was a bit disconcerting, but the labor had progressed so far that there was nothing to do but complete the delivery as a breech presentation.

In any breech presentation there are two terrible things that can happen. The baby's head can be too large to pass through the birth canal without a long period of molding, and the baby' arms can become crossed over the top of its head, which makes delivery impossible. Either situation means big trouble. A big head can often be delivered with the use of special forceps, in which case we would anticipate more or less trauma to the birth canal, and possibly injury to the baby's head. Arms crossed up over the head was an emergency which required the obstetrician to put his hand into the uterus and wipe the forearm and hand on each side downward across the front of the chest and abdomen, which would allow the baby's body to be delivered. Then there would remain the possibility of having trouble getting the baby's un-molded head out, before the baby suffocated.

This time the delivery proceeded normally until the baby's body was born. The head didn't want to drop into the maternal pelvis. With some pressure through the abdominal wall from above, assisted inside the pelvis by some rotation, I managed to get the head to come down into the pelvis. Now it seemed stuck, and time was passing by. If the cord circulation stopped and more than three or four minutes went by, the baby would certainly suffer brain damage. I was just thinking about trying forceps on the after-coming head when I was able to get a finger deep into the baby's mouth and pull its chin firmly down onto its chest. This placed the head in flexion and presented a different diameter to the pelvis, and I was able to extract the head without using great force.

At first the baby was pale and flaccid. He was not breathing. I sucked out the airway thoroughly. I could feel no pulse in the umbilical cord, so I clamped and cut it immediately. I tried the various common maneuvers to stimulate breathing. I snapped my finger at the soles of its feet. I bent the trunk forward, and then hyper-extended it. Still no breaths. I took the baby across the hall to the surgical scrub sinks and ran a little lukewarm water on its body. Then I held its chest under the cold-water spray and was rewarded with a single gasp. Now the nurse arrived with the portable oxygen tank and blew oxygen into the baby's face. Another few seconds in warm water, then cold. Another gasp. Then a third. Then a fourth. With pure oxygen blowing on to its face, the baby began to show a bit of color. Again no more breaths. Trying to keep the baby from becoming hypothermic I held it under the lukewarm water spray most of the time, and intermittently gave it a squirt of cold to make it gasp. I kept this up for about thirty minutes before the baby started to breathe on its own. Now our problem was to keep the baby warm, which we did with a heat lamp, hot water bottles and warm baby blankets. I stayed with him for another hour and a half, and by then he could easily be made to cry. Needless to say I was relieved. We had a live baby with decent color and a fairly good cry, and his mother was recovering nicely.

Now it was my time to worry about this baby. Would he be brain damaged or have other problems related to his difficult birth and resuscitation afterward. Throughout the years I would think about him from time to time, and I actually worried about him until the day, eighteen years later, that I attended the graduation ceremonies at the Eaton Rapids High School. He was the valedictorian of his graduating class!

Soon word was getting around about our practice of allowing fathers into the delivery room, and it was attracting patients from out of town and even out of our territory. There were occasional patients that lived in the shadow of one of the large Lansing hospitals who came to me just to be able to have the father observe the delivery. Then one day I was invited by a Lansing television station to participate in a debate over the desirability of allowing fathers into the delivery room to observe the birth of their offspring. I was alone in speaking for the proposition and opposing me were the formidable presences of the Sister Superior who was the Hospital Administrator for St. Lawrence Hospital, and the obstetrician who was the chief of the Obstetric Department there. I had heard their arguments before.

"Something untoward might happen which would bring a law suit down upon doctor and hospital. The father would get excited and do something dangerous. If something bad happened or there was a bad outcome the father or family would sue. If the mother or baby developed any kind of infection the hospital could be sued for allowing an untrained person into a sterile area. Etc., etc., etc."

My response came from my deep down belief that unless a father actually witnessed the birth of his child, he would never know what an ordeal childbirth actually was, and would remain unaware of the process, which his wife had to endure when she suffered through it. Therefore I believed that the mother had every right to have her husband present. I have often had first time fathers tell me afterward that before actually seeing it, they could not even imagine what their wives went through. I also argued that if something actually did go wrong in the delivery room, and the outcome was less than good, a father, who was present and who witnessed all of the tension and perhaps hectic events connected with such a birth, would better understand the circumstances, and would be less likely to sue, than a father who had spent that time pacing in the lobby only to have the doctor or someone else come out and tell him that he had a dead or deformed baby.

Of course, in the eyes of the St. Lawrence Hospital personnel, and the TV Station people, I lost that debate. However, a little bit more than a year later in a Sunday edition of the Lansing State Journal appeared a full two-page spread with the headline, "ST. LAWRENCE TO ALLOW FATHERS IN THE DELIVERY ROOM." There were large pictures of the Mother Superior and the obstetrican who had debated me, and their quotes about how great it was going to be. Since that time almost all of the hospitals that I know allow fathers in the delivery room. Did I have anything to do with it? I don't know.

In the early days of my practice none of us in the group did Caesarian sections. We called upon Dr. Jason Meads, an obstetrician from Jackson, who would come on short notice and do the surgery in our hospital. He would also come to consult on a difficult labor, and would do the Caesarian section if it were necessary. As I have mentioned before, he would occasionally complete a delivery by doing a version and extraction, which always bothered me, because in it he would turn the baby into a breech presentation and complete the delivery that way.

The operation that Dr. Meads did was the classical Caesarian section, in which the abdomen is opened and then the uterus opened using a long vertical incision through the uterine muscle through which the baby and the placenta (afterbirth) were delivered. The uterus would then contract and the muscular wall would thicken until it was something over two inches thick. There were a lot of blood spaces within this muscle so closure had to be solid in order to assure the control of bleeding. This usually required three layers of catgut sutures in the muscle, and one more to close the peritoneum over it.

The first Caesarian section that Dr. Meads did for me taught me an important lesson that is etched into my mind forever. The operation was not an emergency so it was scheduled in the morning, and was done under spinal anesthesia. Everything went well until about two hours after the surgery, when the patient had considerable vaginal bleeding. I was called and found the uterus to be soft and relaxed. I massaged it through the abdominal wall and got it to contract. This seemed to control the bleeding.

I had the nurse give an extra dose of ergotrate by injection rather than by mouth, as was our custom, but the uterus would not stay contracted, and began to bleed again. More massage got it to contract again, and then a second injection of obstetrical pitocin was given. Before long the uterus relaxed again, and I had to massage it again. I called Dr. Meads, and he suspected right away what the problem was. For postoperative pain I had ordered morphine, and morphine is a notorious uterine relaxing agent. This happened in the days before we had a narcotic antagonist, so I stayed at the bedside for five or six more hours intermittently massaging the uterus to keep it contracted. Finally, after the effect of the morphine had completely worn off, it behaved as it should and remained nicely contracted, while the vaginal flow remained scant and became almost serous. The patient had an uneventful night, and the next day I took a hemoglobinometer up to check her hemoglobin level. I was actually quite shocked to see that it was barely three grams. Normal is twelve or thirteen grams. I considered a blood transfusion, and the trouble I would have accomplishing it. The patient appeared to be in good condition and recovering normally from the surgery, so I prescribed iron by mouth and a high protein diet. When I sent her home a week after the operation her hemoglobin measured six grams, and when she came to the office for her six-week checkup her hemoglobin was normal at a level above thirteen grams.

Another more hectic Caesarian section that Dr. Meads did for me was to a patient who was in her forties. I had seen her earlier when I had first come to town, and had determined that she had severe rheumatic heart disease. She had a huge heart and the typical murmurs of mitral valve disease. The first time I examined her she was already showing early signs of heart failure. Mild diuretics and digitalis helped the heart failure, but I could not be sure that she would not die at anytime soon. When she came to me with increasing complaints of her feet swelling and shortness of breath, it was obvious that her uterus was enlarged. When I heard the little heartbeat inside, I knew for certain that she was pregnant, and I doubted that she could carry the baby to term. I thought she would die first. I considered abortion, and the patient was willing, but abortion was totally illegal unless it could be shown that to carry the pregnancy to term would result in death to the mother. I referred her to a number of specialists, but none would certify that the pregnancy would cause her to die. In the meantime the woman's heart failure was gradually worsening. As she became more bloated with fluid, I was forced into using injectable mercurial diuretics to keep her breathing.

Then sometime near the beginning of her ninth month of pregnancy she arrived at the hospital by ambulance. She was unconscious, wheezing, and had the death rattle in her throat. It looked as if she would truly be dead any minute. The only logical thing to do was to get the baby out to save its life. I called Dr. Meads, and within thirty minutes he was in our operating room in Eaton Rapids. While he was on his way we moved the patient onto the surgical table in the operating room, where we inserted a retention catheter into her bladder to keep it empty. Dr. Herman VanArk was the anesthetist, but the patient was all the while unconscious, and he was continually giving her only pure oxygen to breathe. Dr. Meads was the surgeon and I was the assistant. We had that baby out in record time, and had the patient closed up again in record time. She remained unconscious during the whole operation, and had not received any anesthetic agent at all. We took her downstairs and put her, propped up in bed, into an oxygen tent, and I was surprised and glad to see that her breathing had improved. The next morning she was conscious and seemed comfortable with a minimum of medication. Through her catheter she had lost a tremendous amount of fluid as urine. I restarted her heart medications. The baby was just fine. In a little over a week I was able to send the mother and baby home, and both did well. I know that she lived for a lot of years after that, and I know that she later developed a ventral abdominal hernia through her surgical scar, but eventually I lost track of both mother and baby.

A short time after we started our group practice, the need for more examining room space became apparent, so we had the big front and side porch of the hospital enclosed and heated to create several of them. Our practices grew, especially the obstetric cases. Our patients liked the fact that fathers were allowed in the delivery room, and many of them hailed the advent of saddle block anesthesia as the answer to their difficult labors. All of our hospitalized patients seemed to do well. There were many who entered the hospital with serious conditions who not only survived but also returned to reasonably good health.

CHAPTER IX

STIMSON HOSPITAL CONDEMNED

During the first few years of practice as the Stimson Medical Group we made many small improvements in operations, and were highly satisfied with the way the practice was going. While he was still in the service and stationed in Europe we invited **Dr. Eber B. Sherman**, who was Dr. Bert VanArk's son-in-law, to join our group. I remember talking with him on my office phone. He was in France, and during our conversation he accepted our offer. Dr. Sherman was a graduate of Wayne University Medical School, and later, when he arrived to join us, he fit into our group very well. He turned out to be an excellent physician for our town.

The physicians in the group worked together very well, and from time to time each doctor added new skills to the practice. We soon found that we were taking care of most of the illnesses that occurred in our service area, and it was rarely necessary to refer a case out of town. We took pride in the fact that this was so. We knew that it was beneficial to our patients, because it is always less stressful to have one's illness resolved close to home rather than in some distant big city hospital. We tried diligently to keep things that way, but in the end found it impossible. It was not the will to adequately care for all of our people that failed us; it was lack of capital funds. For example, while we learned how to take and read x-ray tomograms in order to get some kind of a three-dimensional view of a patient's anatomy, this practice became outmoded practically overnight when Computed Axial Tomography became available. These are the famous "CAT Scans" that are now, after many years, still very useful. The early CAT Scanners sold for nearly one million dollars each, which was a sum far beyond our financial resources.

My only real complaint about our practice was that, because our offices were located in the hospital lobby, which never closed, we could not easily break away from our offices to go home at dinnertime. People kept arriving for advice or treatment after regular office hours. However, because we in the group were covering for each other on a schedule, each one of us did manage to have some time off.

Then, without warning, in early 1952 came the threats that eventually put Stimson Hospital out of business. The State and County Health Departments had been inspecting the hospital at least annually for a long time, and each inspection usually resulted in demerits for failure to exactly follow some of the requirements of a few nuisance-type rules. Correcting such deficiencies was neither expensive nor difficult.

One day the County Health Department, which had been inspecting the sanitation in the kitchen more or less regularly, took a culture from the clean dishes in the hospital kitchen, and found that bacteria were present there. This started a process of taking monthly cultures from the clean china and dinnerware that was used to feed the patients and staff, and a month later these cultures were again positive for bacterial contamination. In those days the kitchen served home cooked meals, with food taken directly out of the cook pots on the stove, and placed on the dinnerware on the patient trays. Single portion or single serving packaging was not required, so sanitation practices throughout the entire food service were important.

After the meal the dishes were washed by hand, and after the first citation for germs on the dishes was received, Bernice drastically changed the dishwashing procedure. The dishes, having first been washed with extra strong cleaning solution and water, were then rinsed with scalding hot water from a boiling tea kettle, and allowed to air dry. This did not solve the problem. The next County Health Department inspection turned up bacteria on the dishes again.

Ezra Bohnett was the only male employee on the hospital staff. Besides his janitorial chores, which included mopping and buffing floors, outdoor sweeping and snow shoveling, care of the furnace, and making handyman repairs, Bernice now asked him to look into this problem of bacteria on the dishes. Ezra began by washing the dishes himself, using the strongest cleaning compounds available. The dishwater was so caustic that he had to wear rubber gloves. Then he soaked the dishes in strong bleach solution for a while. Then he let them air dry. Still the next inspection turned up bacteria on the dishes once more. Ezra changed the cleaning compounds and the washing process again, and had the cook and meal servers wear surgical masks. Again this didn't solve the problem, and after three or four alterations of the dishwashing methods, Ezra was almost beside himself with guilt, thinking it was he who might be the source of the germs.

It so happened that I was in my office the next time that the health inspector arrived to inspect the hospital, and knowing about the problem with the "dirty" dishes, I decided to accompany her on her rounds. I had seen this woman a number of times before, and had the impression that she wasn't exactly brilliant. She kept talking all the while that we were inspecting the patient floors upstairs. When we got to the kitchen down in the basement, she hardly looked at anything, but went right to the job of taking cultures from the dishes. To take them she used sterile cotton tipped swabs, which came in sterile glass tubes. After wiping each swab around on a dish, she put each into a second sterile tube containing a small amount of culture medium. She would hold a dish or other item up to the light, pull the swab from its tube, rub the cotton tip around on the dish, and then put the swab into the second tube containing the sterile culture medium. She was not wearing gloves or a surgical mask, and as she was obtaining the swabs, she talked constantly. As she moved the swab tip about on a plate I could see the saliva drops spray out of her mouth onto the plate. Here, obviously was the cause for the whole series of bad culture reports!!!!

"Wait a minute!" I said, "I've been watching you take your cultures. You can't seem to keep your mouth shut long enough to take a proper culture. I've been watching the shower of your saliva spray on to that plate several times while you were swabbing it for the culture."

She bristled in defense, but I was disturbed, and continued to upbraid her, telling her, among other things, that I thought she didn't have enough common sense to be a health inspector.

"From now on," I almost shouted, "I expect cultures to be taken properly, and I expect correct, honest culture reports in the future."

We immediately returned to the old dishwashing system in which the dishes were washed with soap and water, rinsed with water, and air-dried, and we didn't have any more positive cultures from our kitchen.

No sooner had we resolved this problem, than a second and larger threat to the hospital's existence arrived in the form of a more complete than usual inspection of the hospital building by an inspector from the State Fire Marshall's office. Up until that time the State Fire Marshall's office had made some irregular and more or less haphazard inspections, but this time we were hit with a list of major deficiencies, and given a time limit within which we had to comply. The main points of the deficiency list were that (1) we must install an automatic fire sprinkler system in all rooms of the building, (2) we must enclose the stairwell from the basement to the top floor with fire resistant material and install fire doors on all exits and entrances to it. There was also a long list of other minor, less expensive requirements, which I don't exactly remember now. The time allowed to comply with these requirements was relatively short. It was urgent that we decide what to do!

First we contacted some friends in the building and contracting business, and from them received rough estimates of what such a project would cost. All of the estimates were above $100,000. This amount or more had to be spent for the required alterations to a building for which we had paid substantially less than $25,000 only some four years earlier. Raising that amount of money might have been possible, but it would have strained the financial resources of our medical group, and the economics of doing it didn't make sense to me. I thought it would be throwing good money into a doubtful project, and that the result would be prone to further attacks by the governmental powers. Such money would be much better spent on a new building, on a larger plot of ground.

The gravity of the situation struck me. The other doctors in our group felt about as I did, and we decided that this was a decision that should be placed before the citizens of the hospital's service area.

CHAPTER X

THE BIRTH OF A NEW HOSPITAL

Because I was a member of the local Kiwanis Club, my colleagues asked me to present our problems with the State Fire Marshal to the Kiwanis Club of Eaton Rapids. The Kiwanians Program Committee granted my request to do this, and allowed me to have the entire program at the next meeting.

A large number of people were present, and in my talk I told them about the State Fire Marshall's requirements, our cost estimates, and the pros and cons of renovating the hospital building, or closing it and not having a hospital in Eaton Rapids at all. I offered my opinion that the cost of renovating the old hospital building was prohibitive, especially when comparing it to what might be obtained for the same money, if it were used for a part of the cost of a new building.

Much to the credit of those Kiwanians, the club decided to sponsor an open town meeting to present the problem to the public, and within a short time a well attended area wide citizens meeting was held. An unusually large and representative crowd attended this meeting. As was the case in many small town and rural areas, there were, in general, two schools of thought about public projects. The old guard, the people who were well established in the status quo, was generally conservative, and disliked spending money. At the other end of the spectrum were the younger go-getters and people still working up to where they would some day be satisfied with the status quo. I presented the hospital's problems and the State Fire Marshall's demands for correcting them, and emphasized that these demands had to be met in order to keep the hospital open and running. I presented the estimates for what the work was likely to cost, and added my opinion that paying for remodeling was no bargain. Members of the audience were invited to speak and express their opinions, and during this time I heard most of the objections to doing anything at all, including the one, "Why should we pay for a workplace for the doctors?" I explained that the hospital was central to our practices and very important to us, and if there were no hospital in town, the three of us would probably move to an area that had a hospital. After considerable discussion with back and forth questions and answers, it appeared that the consensus of the group was to have a fund drive to remodel the condemned Stimson Hospital Building.

Then something happened that almost instantly changed the tenor of the whole meeting. A woman --- I believe it was Mrs. Ruth McNamara--- stood up and said emphatically,

"There is absolutely no reason in the world why this town cannot build a new hospital!!"

This produced some muffled cheers, and shouts of agreement. I could sense the enthusiasm build, and the meeting finally ended with a resolution to have a fund drive to build a new hospital for Eaton Rapids. The very next week the first "bake sale" for the benefit of the new hospital was held.

This decision by the Citizen's Committee to build a new hospital started a significant train of events, which occurred in quick succession. Richard Robinson, then an Eaton Rapids attorney, donated his services to write Articles of Incorporation, which established the new hospital as a legal entity. Lawyer Robinson later became Judge Robinson, and sat for 16 years as Circuit Court judge for the district which included Eaton Rapids. The name chosen for the hospital was EATON RAPIDS COMMUNITY HOSPITAL. At my insistence the Articles of Incorporation stipulated that no member of any of the healing professions could serve as a director. My purpose was to counteract any idea, that the public might have, that it was building a new hospital for the benefit of the doctors, or that doctors would have any direct financial control over it. A Board of Directors was elected. One of its first acts was the adoption of the Articles of Incorporation, and the election of officers of the board. Lawrence McNamara, the local Oldsmobile dealer, was elected its President, and he worked very, very hard to make the dream of having a new hospital come true.

Land ---a whole city block on Main Street at the South city limits--- was donated by G. Elmer McArthur, a prominent Eaton Rapids attorney, with the stipulation that the donated land must be turned over to the City of Eaton Rapids if the site were ever to become anything but a hospital.

The Hospital Fund Drive began under the direction of the new board of directors. The doctors and several other prominent people of the area donated immediately. Others signed pledges. People volunteered to go house to house to explain the new hospital concept and collect money and pledges for it. Organizations scheduled fund raising events for the benefit of the hospital. A committee was formed to solicit donations from commercial businesses both inside and outside of our hospital area. It appeared that an overwhelming majority of the people in the hospital service area was solidly behind the project.

Meanwhile a number of people, myself included, who were close to the project, began to busy themselves with the planning of the actual construction. It was important to us that the building should be of high grade, lasting construction, and also that we should not overpay for it. With an eye toward saving construction expense and making the hospital's funds go farther, we did not hire an architect. Instead I made floor plan drawings, patterning the patient rooms after those in the hospitals being used by the Mayo Clinic in Rochester, Minnesota. I had been very favorably impressed with them when I had visited my brother, Richard K. Meinke, M.D., while he was serving his residency in surgery there. The electric system was drawn up by the electricians of the Nicholas Electric firm in Eaton Rapids. It included provision for a stand-by electric generator to be used when there was a power failure. Balcom Plumbing, a local firm, was involved in laying out the plumbing. Although the building would be connected to city water and sewer, the plan also called for a large bore well to be drilled on the property and connected in such a way that it could become an "on call" water supply for the whole hospital if needed in an emergency. After the building was finished and in use, a local well driller named Edward Cords donated his time, supplies and equipment to drill and connect a 12-inch well for the hospital.

Mr. McArthur, the man who had donated the land, had a keen interest in concrete and concrete structures. He said his experience had included building a lot of curb and sewer construction in Eaton Rapids. Following many of his suggestions, the board agreed upon a concrete and brick building, which had the advantage of being inherently fireproof. The outside walls were of concrete block, insulated with a thick layer of Styrofoam, and then covered on the above ground surfaces with ordinary brick. There was much discussion about whether or not to build a basement, and because basement space was the least expensive space we could build, we decided to have one. This decision turned out to be most fortunate because eventually all of the basement space was needed and used. The inside walls were also constructed of concrete block where weight bearing was needed, and cinder block where weight bearing was not needed. Here and there, and for later additions, metal lath and drywall plaster were used. The main floor and the roof were constructed of commercially pre-cast concrete slabs with the trade name, Flexicore. They were really concrete beams, about one foot wide, six inches thick, and containing three hollow tubes running their full length. They also contained steel reinforcement rods for their full length and had both great strength and rigidity. They were laid closely together, side by side upon the bearing walls of the building to form a strong, solid plane surface. The basement had the usual four-inch concrete floor. On the first floor the Flexicore was covered with a two-inch layer of concrete over which carpeting and various types of floor tile were eventually installed. The ceilings inside were the smooth lower surfaces of the Flexicore beams, painted or otherwise treated. The Flexicore beams, which made up the roof, were also covered with a thin layer of concrete. Then six inches of insulation were laid upon it, and over that a built up flat layer of roofing was installed. Heavy insulation was needed because the building was to be heated by electricity, which was not the cheapest energy that could have been used. Other fuels, however, would require air ducts and central heat generators (furnaces or boilers), which would have added significantly to the cost of the building.

As soon as it appeared that enough money for the project was being donated, a general contractor who would go along with the piecemeal plans that were available was hired. It was a young firm from Jackson, Michigan, the name of which has escaped me. The people of this firm were most cooperative and worked enthusiastically, as did some of the local trades people who also worked on the building. Cooperation was great. As problems arose, minds came together to create solutions. After a set of plans had been approved by both the State Health Department and the State Fire Marshall, the construction began during warm weather with the digging out of the shallow basement. Mr. McArthur, who had donated the land for the hospital, involved himself with the cement work. I was frequently consulted about the medical aspects of the building, which included such things as the placement of light fixtures, sinks, cabinets, etc., and the piping of oxygen from a central source to the head of each hospital bed.

The construction of the surgical wing of the hospital was special because of the many extra regulations that applied to it. I researched not only the regulations, but also many construction methods and materials, and some of the ideas I turned up were included in the construction. Regulations required that the air in the surgery must be re-circulated every two minutes with the continuous addition of 20% by volume of fresh, outside air. This required some type of a furnace system with a fan, air ducts, and filters. The filters were required to remove dust particles and bacteria from the air, a requirement that was practically impossible to achieve with any kind of furnace filter, or combinations of such filters, and still allow for enough circulating air volume. The room must also have a positive air pressure, so that "contaminated" air from another part of the hospital could not be sucked into it. This required that a bigger volume of air had to be blown into the room than could leave it through the return air ducts. The addition of the 20% outside air achieved this requirement nicely. The return air duct system was so sized that it could not accommodate a greater volume of exhaust air than the volume of re-circulated air being blown into the room, so the extra volume of outside air injected into the room served to raise the air pressure inside. Of course most of this extra pressure was lost to "air leaks" from the room, and to outward gushes of room air whenever the door was opened. When the swinging doors to the surgery were finally installed, one could see that, when they were closed, air pressure in the room kept them slightly ajar as the extra, added air escaped from the room.

Another consideration was the lighting in the surgery. The large floodlights especially made for use in surgical operating rooms were so big that if one were to be hung on a ceiling of ordinary height, it would reach at least half way to the floor. For this reason we designed the surgical wing to be one and one half stories high, with the operating room utilizing that entire height. The rest of the surgical wing consisted of a sterilization and supply room, a doctors' dressing room, a nurses' dressing room and the hospital emergency room, all of which had about one half of a normal floor height above them as an attic.

The floor of the operating room was also special. It had to conduct electricity freely in order to carry away static electricity, which may build up on people or equipment as they moved around or were used in the room. People entering the surgery had to wear special conductive shoes, or shoe covers made of conductive material which had a special flap that had to be tucked into ones street shoes and under the sole of the foot in order to conduct electricity to the conductive floor. These regulations were necessary because some of the anesthesia substances that were commonly in use were highly flammable, and there was the constant danger of a spark of static electricity from someone's body causing a severe and dangerous explosion. Theoretically the chest of a patient under anesthesia and breathing in ether or cyclopropane and oxygen was a human bomb, which could be set off by a spark of static electricity. For our floor we chose vinyl tiles into which conductive substances had been incorporated. These tiles were laid over thin copper strips on the floor with cement that also contained conductive material. The copper strips were all connected to a large ground wire, designed to carry electricity off into the ground. Thus, anyone or anything coming into the operating room holding a charge of static electricity (from the shuffling of feet or whatever) would have the electricity immediately and safely discharged through this floor system, and would no longer be a hazard.

Although the rest of the hospital building was to be heated with baseboard electric heaters, the operating room could not be heated in this manner because of the air exchange regulations.

As the heat source we chose a small gas furnace installed in the attic space above and adjacent to the operating room. Access to it was through a large trap door in the ceiling of the hallway outside of the surgery. Its duct system supplied warm air directly to the operating room, and a return air system of ducts returned the room air back to the furnace. Just before the return air arrived back to be re-circulated through the furnace an accessory duct system with a volume regulator in it allowed the necessary 20 percent of outside to be added to the main circulating stream of air. After this mixture of outside and re-circulated air passed through the heating chamber of the furnace, but before it entered the operating room, it had to pass through an automatic humidifier which relied upon the evaporation of water, and through an electronic filter, which was a relatively new filtering device designed to remove even the smallest of particles from the air. It consisted of two sets of conductive metal plates, held rigidly in place, interdigitating with each other, but nowhere touching each other. These plates were charged with a direct current electric circuit, so one set of plates became positively charged and the other became negatively charged. When the air stream passed through between the charged plates, all particles, depending upon their natural, inherent static electric charge, would be drawn to one or the other set of plates and cling there. (*It is a natural law of static electricity that like charges repel and opposite charges attract each other.*) Any particles which were neutral (*carried no charge, were neither positive or negative*) would brush against one of the charged plates, and either pick up an electron from the plate to become negatively charged, or give up an electron to the plate to become positively charged. It would then be instantly attracted to the plate which carried its opposite charge and cling there. No matter how small the particle might be, this system could pick it out of the air without difficulty. It was an ideal system for cleaning operating room air, and maintenance was simple. First the electricity was turned off. The particles on the plates, which then were no longer attracted to them, were washed off with jets of water installed in the air chamber which held the plates, and the dirty water went down the drain. I kept patting myself on the back, quite content that we had found the best system possible.

However, when the hospital building was nearly complete, and the heating and air handling system was in operation, we had an inspection by the State Health Department. The inspector disallowed our electronic filter. I explained it to him in much the same way, but much greater detail, as I have explained it here, but he still wouldn't approve it, saying that he needed to see blueprints. I showed him the literature that we had accumulated and the specifications for the equipment, which came with the manufacturer's installation instructions, but he hardly looked at them. Finally I said to him,

"Let me take you up into the attic and demonstrate the equipment. I'll show you how it operates."

He replied, "I'm not going up there. It wouldn't do any good. I wouldn't know what I was looking at. I'm AN ENGINEER. I need blueprints!"

Therefore, before we were allowed to open the new hospital we had to have the electronic filter removed, and have an old fashioned furnace filter box with changeable fiber filters installed. What a waste! Little did I know then that this would not be the last time I would be compelled to go head to head with inept, incompetent regulatory personnel.

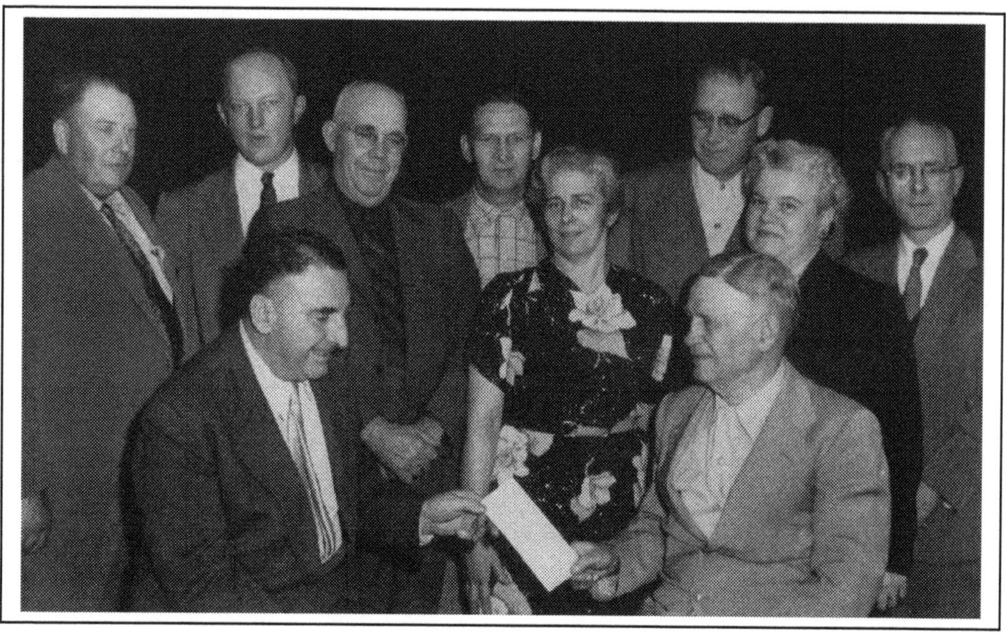

The Board of Directors of the new Eaton Rapids Community Hospital shortly before it opened. Included in the picture is the author, Dr. Meinke, who had been named Medical Director for the new Hospital, but was not a member of the Board. Pictured are: (standing from left) Herbert VanAken, Dr. Albert Meinke, Jr., Leo Benjamin, Ray Hocott, Bernice Bowman, John (Jack) Davidson, Eva Chadwick, and Kenneth Williams (Treasurer). Seated are Lawrence McNamara (President) and G. Elmer McArthur.

The very first Board of directors elected by the donors to the hospital included Roland Topliff, who was replaced later by John Davidson. Before the hospital actually opened Ray Hocott was replaced by George Miller of the Miller Dairy Farms.

CHAPTER XI

THE TRANSITION

Construction on the new hospital building ran on through the summer and fall. It continued slowly throughout the winter, and by late spring of 1957 the project was nearing completion. We had to make plans to close Stimson Hospital and open the new one. As owners of Stimson, we (the doctors) agreed to donate free of charge all of the Stimson Hospital furnishings and equipment to the new hospital. This included everything from the operating room, delivery room, nursery, hospital pharmacy, kitchen and all patient rooms.

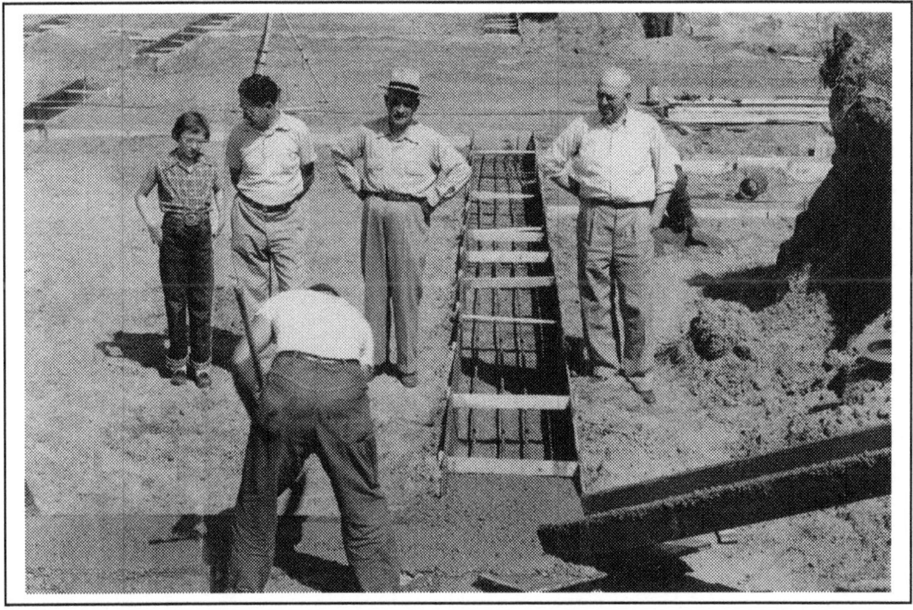

Footings being poured for the new Eaton Rapids Community Hospital building. Shown supervising the cement work is G. Elmer McArthur flanked on the left by Ray Hocott and his daughter, Nancy. On the right also watching the work is Leo Benjamin.

The Veterans of Foreign Wars National Home operated an orphanage for the children and widows of veterans. They had a lovely campus about three miles from downtown Eaton Rapids, with numerous individual brick homes. Also included was a hospital, which was well equipped, but not used much. The doctors in our group regularly visited to see sick children there, but did not admit patients there. Except for a campus nurse, the VFW Hospital had no regular administration or staff. The Veterans of Foreign Wars organization agreed to donate its surgical equipment and x-ray machine to the new hospital. Their x-ray machine was also a Picker X-Ray machine, which was somewhat higher powered and newer than the one we had at Stimson Hospital. So the machine from the VFW Hospital was moved and installed in the new hospital well before the hospital was scheduled to open, and we continued to use the one in Stimson Hospital as our office machine until we eventually moved out of that building. Later the machine from Stimson was traded in on a new x-ray machine for the new hospital, and then there were two in use there.

In the meantime, Bernice Bowman, who had operated Stimson Hospital by herself, and then later operated it for us as its owners, stated that she wished to retire. She didn't want to become the administrator of the new hospital, but she would gladly make herself available for help and advice to whomever was hired to that position. So the board advertised for a new hospital administrator.

Response to their advertisements was not large, and a number of the people who applied were obviously not qualified for the position. After screening what there was, the board decided to interview one of them, a nurse who was working in the Veterans' Administration Hospital at Fort Custer in Battle Creek, Michigan. I cannot now remember her name, but I was one of the three people who went to Battle Creek to interview her. She was a bit past her prime in years, but had good nursing credentials and seemed to be a business-like person. In the end we hired her to be the first hospital administrator of the EATON RAPIDS COMMUNITY HOSPITAL, and Bernice spent time helping her after she arrived on the job.

In the weeks before the new hospital building was ready for occupancy, the hospital board experienced some anxious times about paying for it. It appeared that enough donations and pledges had been received to cover the expenditures, but there was always the worry that some certain percent of the pledges would not be made good. The board had already spent much time and effort to see to it that all of its money was wisely spent, and that none was squandered.

During one of these "expense" discussions I expressed the opinion that before the building was ready for occupancy, over $260,000 would have been spent. Leo Benjamin, who had also served on the city council, and whom I considered to be somewhat of a politician, or at least a "good old boy," made a bet with me that the project would cost less than that. If it turned out to be more than $260,000, he would buy me a new hat. If it turned out to be less, I would buy him a new hat. About two weeks before the project was finished it appeared that the cost would indeed be approximately $240,000. I owed Leo a hat!

Shortly before the new hospital was to open, the Kiwanis Club scheduled an evening banquet to celebrate that imminent event. Numerous local dignitaries including Leo Benjamin were invited, so I thought that this would be a good time to make good my bet with him, and pay up. I didn't want to pick out a hat for him, so I decided to give him a gift certificate. I went downtown to Vic Alt's Mens' Wear Store, and told Vic about my bet with Leo. Vic suggested a gift certificate offering being made by the Stetson Co., a famous hat maker, in which the gift certificate was wrapped up in a miniature hatbox, which also contained a miniature Stetson hat. I paid for one of the higher priced hats, and took the miniature home, intending to give it to Leo at the Kiwanis celebration.

When the time came for the banquet to begin, the room in which it was being held was crowded. Leo was a hospital board member and was seated at the head table, but by the time I had worked my way through the crowd to his place, he had gone to the rest room. So I left the little hatbox by his placecard with a note saying that this was payment for our bet. I did not sit near Leo that evening, and I was not a part of the program, nor did I see Leo during the exodus after the end of the ceremonies. However, before I left for home one of Leo's dining companions reported to me that Leo had returned to the table, looked a my note, opened the tiny hat box and took out the tiny hat. Then he turned livid, hopping-mad that I had "stiffed" him out of a good hat. Only after he found the gift certificate did he settle down. I believe that he got his hat, but I cannot recall a single time that Leo has spoken to me since that day. Sometimes I wonder about that?

On the Sunday afternoon before the new hospital was to open and admit patients, dedication ceremonies were held on the hospital grounds. The weather was nice and there were many people present. The speeches were short. I don't remember that I was asked to speak, but I do remember that I was given the honor of cutting the ceremonial ribbon at the entrance to the hospital.

The next day we made the move from Stimson Hospital. It was done all at one time, since there was plenty of volunteer help. Both funeral directors in town volunteered the use of their ambulances to transfer the patients the one mile or so to the new location. Local movers and other people with trucks volunteered to move furniture, equipment and furnishings. Empty beds in the old building were moved and made up in the new hospital to receive patients as they were transferred, until, first all patients and, finally, all beds had been transferred.

Eaton Rapids Community Hospital was open for business. Stimson Hospital no longer existed.

CHAPTER XII

EATON RAPIDS COMMUNITY HOSPITAL

The transition from the old to the new hospital had gone smoothly. The first birth in the new hospital was an unexpected one, because the baby was born a month or so prematurely to one of my patients, a Mrs. Canfield. Mother and baby did well.

It did not take long for me to become accustomed to the new surroundings, and it was a pleasure to work with everything located on one floor. We now had a real emergency room with its own separate entrance, and a nurse on duty. The doctors took emergency call in an agreed-upon rotation, and the system seemed to work well.

The summer and fall of 1957 passed uneventfully, and I was beginning to feel quite comfortable about everything, when our hospital administrator, the nurse from Battle Creek, told us that she wanted to resign. She agreed to remain for a while, however, to allow time for us to find her replacement. No one seemed very upset about this, perhaps because no one felt that, during her tenure as administrator, she had established a decent rapport with employees or patients.

Once again the recruitment process was set in motion, and advertisements announcing that the position was open were placed nationwide in various appropriate publications. Our previous experience with such advertising had not produced much, and we were quite uncertain about finding competent leadership for our new hospital.

Among the few applications we received in answer to our ads, one stood out from the rest, and we decided to interview this applicant. He was still serving in the U.S. Army at Fort Bragg, North Carolina, where he was in the Medical Corps as a laboratory technician in the Station Hospital.

After some correspondence and a few phone calls we arranged to meet and interview him on a definite, specific date at Fort Bragg. Lawrence McNamara (the local Oldsmobile dealer), George Miller (of Miller Dairy Farms) and I agreed to go. The plan was for us to leave Eaton Rapids in my car early in the morning on the day before the interview, and drive to the airport in Akron, Ohio, where George Miller had just had his airplane put through one of its routine interval inspections and servicings. The plane would be ready for us to fly from there to Fort Bragg, where we should arrive well before dark.

When we arrived in Akron, the plane was still being serviced, and was not quite ready. After about an hour's delay, the servicing was finished and we climbed aboard. George went through all of the moves and checks required to get started, and we taxied out to the starting point on the runway. The tower gave permission to take off. Everything was normal until we were about 300 to 400 feet in the air, when one of the plane's hydraulic lines started to spray hydraulic fluid into the cabin. George turned in a circle, told the tower he was going to land, and brought the plane down on a runway without any further problem. However, as the plane was turning to land, I kept hearing the tower warn George that he was about to stall. I knew that when a plane stalls in flight it could fall like a stone and crash, so I was much relieved when we were on the ground again.

George then made the decision not to try to fly the plane again until it had been thoroughly rechecked once more, and since this would take a considerable amount of time, we decided to take turns at the wheel, and drive on to Fort Bragg. We expected to reach it late in the evening, but the trip turned out to be most tedious. Floods had caused some of the rivers along our route to overflow, and we passed through several places where we were compelled to drive slowly because there was water standing on the roadways. At one point we were not allowed to drive through, so we had to backtrack and choose an alternate route to get to where we wanted to go. We finally arrived at the outskirts of Fort Bragg at about 3:30 a.m., and were able to rent a motel room in which we managed to get some sleep.

Up again at dawn, we checked out of the motel, and after some breakfast, were at the gate at Fort Bragg. We were admitted, guided to the station hospital, and, once inside, found the laboratory without difficulty.

The man we had come to interview was there, working alone on some laboratory tests that had been ordered by the hospital medical staff. His name was **Edward McRee**. After introductions and some initial conversation, we learned that his parents lived in Oklahoma, and that he had grown up there. He was married. His first child was on the way, and would probably be born before his service in the Army was finished. He was trained in medical laboratory technology, but had no experience at all in hospital management. He was polite, and apologized for the circumstance that he had to continue some of his laboratory work while we talked. He gave direct and straightforward answers to our questions, and I soon noted that he seemed to know more about the laboratory tests he was performing than one would get from just following an instruction manual. We had barely started our interview, and I was already convinced that this was our man!!!

Now George Miller and Larry McNamara took over, and asked more questions, most of which seemed to be related to business practices. When they were finished, the three of us discussed the interview privately.

We had all been favorably impressed, and I felt strongly that we could never find a more suitable candidate for the position. Here was a young man with high intelligence, excellent deportment, a good personality and an obvious desire to do the job, but who had no experience in hospital administration. We had a new small hospital, with a scanty operational track record, and we were looking for someone to put our hospital into good operating condition and run it well. The two were made for each other, and I said so immediately. The other two men were a bit skeptical because of the candidate's young age, but I didn't think that mattered. This young man was capable, and I knew it!

My memory of what happened next is now a bit dim, but I believe that we offered to hire Ed on the spot, but he, showing practical good sense, said that he had no idea where Eaton Rapids was, and that he would like to see both the town and the hospital before he could make up his mind to accept our offer. So we arranged a trip to Eaton Rapids for him, and hoped to be able to employ him when he came to see us. It was only the middle of the morning when we left Fort Bragg, and all three of us had the feeling that we had accomplished something important. Subsequent events over many years proved that, indeed, we had! We drove all day, and arrived back in Eaton Rapids that evening.

Ed did come to Eaton Rapids about two weeks later, and stayed in the guest lodge at the VFW National Home. Before he left, he accepted our offer to become Administrator of Eaton Rapids Community Hospital. I believe that everyone concerned had good feelings about it.

Because Ed could not come to work for us until his stint in the Army had ended, we had to wait upon his arrival for several weeks. During the interval Ed's wife, Jan, gave birth to their first son at the Station Hospital in Fort Bragg. Our now temporary nurse/administrator was not happy about the delay in Ed's arrival, but she did stay on the job, and, with increasing amounts of help from Bernice Bowman, the hospital operated satisfactorily. I am sure that Bernice was also of great help to Ed in his early days immediately after he arrived on the job.

One day, soon after Ed had started to work, he and I sat in the dining area of the hospital kitchen for over an hour, and figured out a budget for the hospital to guide its next year of operation. Ed wrote out the budget, and I offered estimates and opinions about individual budget items. A year later we sat in the same place and repeated the exercise. I was elated to find out that the hospital operation, for the year just ended, had turned out to be within pennies of that first budget! To me this was a good omen for the future. The next few years did go well.

Gradually some profound changes from the old way of practicing medicine came about. Under Ed the hospital laboratory was expanded to offer more tests and services, and medical technicians were hired. Medical record keeping was improved and upgraded, and a department was established to keep the medical records filed and organized. Dictation service was begun, so the doctors could save time by dictating medical histories, operative reports, and other documents. The typists hired were not trained in medical terms, and had to learn on the job as they went along. At first some of the spellings of words in those early documents were fantastic, but it was not long before our typists became proficient with medical terms, and the reports then were excellent.

Arrangements were made with several Lansing pathologists for having autopsies done when needed, and later with the Pathology Department at Ingham Medical Hospital to do the pathologic tissue examinations on all tissues removed in our hospital.

A separate X-ray Department was begun with Charles O. Long, M.D. as the first radiologist of the hospital at its head. Dr. Long's group operated in Ingham Medical Hospital, and soon included, Carl West, M.D., Arthur Budden, M.D. and Thomas Payne, M.D. One of these radiologists came to our hospital once a week, and later twice a week, to do fluoroscopy examinations, and to read all of the x-ray films taken during the preceding week. The hospital also hired x-ray technicians, and we doctors no longer took our own x-rays. I remember occasionally threatening to do so, but the technicians made themselves so available that I never did expose another x-ray film. We still had to read most of our films ourselves, especially the ones taken for emergency cases, but we were now supported, and when necessary, corrected in our x-ray interpretations by a board certified radiologist.

After Ed had headed our hospital for about five years, one of the large hospitals in Lansing began a reorganization. This hospital had had a modest beginning as the Ingham County (Tuberculosis) Sanitarium. Then with a number of chest specialists and chest surgeons on its staff, it began to be known as the Ingham Chest Hospital. Eventually it moved into the field of Open Heart Surgery. Now its board of directors wanted to establish a full-service, complete medical hospital, and asked our Ed McRee to be its administrator. No one wanted to see Ed leave, but the entire hospital board and most of the hospital staff urged Ed to accept the offer. It could be the chance of a lifetime for him.

Ed did leave us to accept the position, and became the administrator of Ingham Medical Hospital, but the circumstances of his leaving were not ordinary. First he recommended that we hire our head laboratory technician, Charles Cartwright, as his replacement, and after the change was made, he coached Charles and made himself available for any needed assistance. He and his family did not move out of Eaton Rapids. Ingham Medical Hospital was about twelve miles away, and Ed commuted daily. His children went to Eaton Rapids Schools, and his family attended church in Eaton Rapids. Ed remained as head of the Ingham Medical system until he retired, but during all of those many years, and now long after his retirement, he has remained interested in almost everything going on in Eaton Rapids. Ed served on the Board of Education of the Eaton Rapids Public Schools, and also on the board of the Eaton Rapids Community Hospital, and was actively involved in its metamorphosis into the present day EATON RAPIDS MEDICAL CENTER. He still sits on the Medical Center Board.

As the director of Ingham Medical Hospital, Ed soon began to make a name for himself. Eventually he became well known all over the state, and, in time, achieved national recognition. When I think back upon that trip we made to interview him at Fort Bragg, I remember my first impression of Ed. I am proud of him, and very pleased that my very early evaluation had been entirely correct.

I don't know exactly how much help and advice Ed gave to Chuck Cartwright, but our hospital continued to run well. Chuck was well liked and seemed to have the ability to get things done without unnecessarily antagonizing people, which is a good trait for an administrator to have. It wasn't long before the Eaton County Long Term Medical Care Facility in Charlotte asked him to become their administrator. Chuck accepted the offer, and also chose to keep his family in Eaton Rapids while he commuted to and from this job. We had to find another administrator.

I was involved in the hiring of the next two administrators of our hospital. The first was John Williams, who had grown up in the Clare, Michigan area, was married and had experience in accounting. After him we hired David VanDeVusse from southwest Michigan, who had some public relations experience. Under trying circumstances, both men did well in their management of the hospital. Both were plagued by governmental regulators to the point of absurdity. For example, when the hospital first opened, it was required to file only a few documents with the government, and pass an annual sanitation inspection in order to stay open. By the time that VanDeVusse's tenure had ended the number of inspections and filing of reports had risen to eighteen or nineteen. It was difficult and expensive to comply with all of the regulations, and partly because of the myriad of regulations it had to obey, the hospital appeared to be heading down the road to financial difficulty.

Once again Ed McRee stepped in to help. Our hospital had already affiliated itself with Ingham Medical Hospital in purchasing agreements and shared services in order to save money. Now Ed proposed sharing administrative services as well. As a result James Miller, who was on the management staff of Ingham Medical Hospital was sent to become the administrator of our hospital. He remained on the Ingham Medical payroll, and our hospital paid Ingham a monthly fee to cover his salary. This connected our Eaton Rapids Community Hospital to the same excellent management expertise that had done so well for the development of Ingham Medical Hospital.

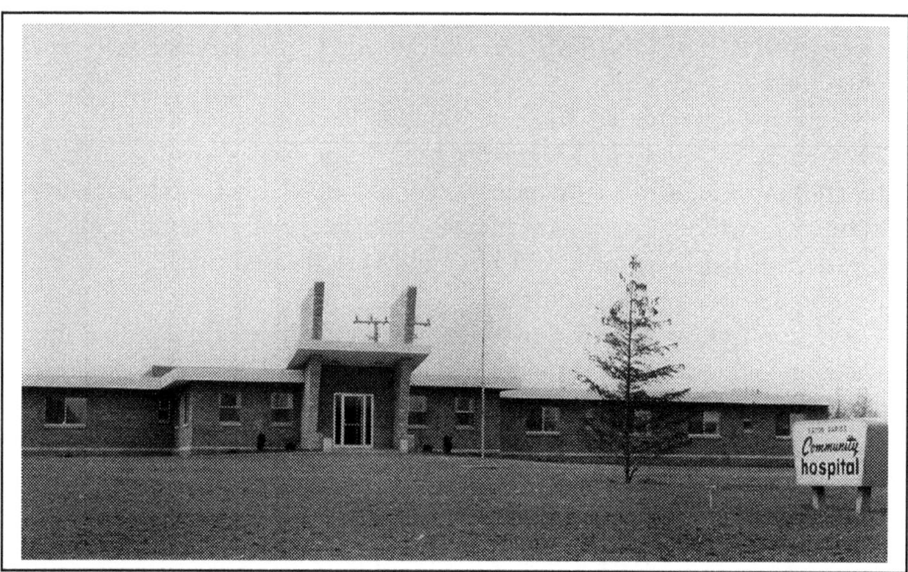

This picture of the Eaton Rapids Community Hospital was taken a short time after Ed McRee arrived to become its administrator. The spruce tree in the foreground was the first bit of landscaping that was donated to the hospital. In the center is the main entrance, and to the right (not completely shown) there were several more patient rooms and a sunroom containing four beds. Eventually this main entrance became the entrance to the emergency room, and it is still a part of the emergency suite today.

CHAPTER XIII

REGULATOR PROBLEMS

During the planning and development which led to the creation of our Eaton Rapids Community Hospital, we were aware that some Federal monies were available for such projects, and we reviewed some of the application processes required in order to obtain them. All were complicated, and included conditions which smacked of government interference, so we did not submit any applications.

Our hospital was built without any government money, and we believed that the government would not bother us, but would allow us to run our hospital in the best interests of the people we served. Now we all know that this belief was entirely wrong! We should have recognized the clues that the regulators had given us in their directives to Stimson Hospital before we finally closed it.

As the years went by, different individual inspectors, came and went, and all seemed to find something wrong to report. While most of the deficiencies were aggravating, they were usually small, and were easy and not very expensive to correct. However, right from the beginning there was a problem with the corridor doors in our new building. The building code required that each patient room must open into a corridor at a point from which an outside exit could be reached within a definite, limited number of feet, and that all of the corridors needed to have doors that closed off segments of corridor containing a limited length. These regulations were intended to allow for getting patients out of the building in case of fire, and closing off the section which was burning from the rest of the hospital. Our outside exits and corridor doors were all properly placed, so the regulators concentrated their efforts on the doors themselves.

Corridor doors were expected to be in pairs and to swing open freely in both directions. Ours did. There had to be a small glass window in each door, placed so that anyone trying to open it could be sure that no one was coming through from the opposite direction. Ours complied. The doors had to be of solid, not hollow, construction. Ours were.

First, after a number of inspections in which the doors were not cited, an inspector found that the windows in the doors were too small. The doors had to be taken down, larger windows installed, and then re-hung. The next year the windows were still too small, and the process was repeated. Next, after some time had passed, double strength glass was no good. It had to be replaced with plate glass. Next, plate glass was no good and had to be replaced with glass into which chicken wire mesh had been fused. After a few more years this glass had to be replaced with plain plate glass again. Then, when the front area of the hospital was remodeled and an addition was put on to the building, the kitchen was moved into the basement, the old lobby was incorporated into what became the new emergency suite, and a new lobby was added. After the plans had been approved by all regulatory agencies, the addition was built, but it did not pass the first fire marshal inspection because it didn't have an automatic steel fire door in the basement between the new construction and the old. The costs of all of this regulation quickly approached the amount of money spent on the entire original hospital construction.

A major problem arose when the State Health Department objected to the fact that there were regular patient beds located on the hallway which ran from the main nursing station, past the post partum maternity rooms and the newborn nursery, to them. The labor and delivery rooms were across the hall from the nursery, and the newborns as well as the mothers had to cross this "tainted" hall soon after each birth. To serve the labor room we had already constructed a new entrance, which came off of the hallway across from the emergency room, so that the new mother-to-be did not need to walk through any "contaminated" area to get there. Now, according to the Health Department, the only solution would be to add an obstetrical wing to the building, and use the space that the obstetrics department was now using for other purposes.

There was room for an extension at the south end of the building, where there was originally a sunroom ward with four beds. If the building extension were to be angled slightly, the open angle would allow ample space for the construction of the required outside entrance. Plans were drawn which included a new emergency room below the obstetric floor, and an elevator so that stretcher patients could be carried up and down.

The plan allowed the obstetric wing to be completely closed off from the rest of the hospital by double doors. The wing included a labor room, and, across the hall, a delivery room with adjacent scrub sinks, a supply room, staff dressing rooms, a nursing station, a newborn nursery, and four post partum rooms. Financing was arranged. Permission was received from the State Health Department to proceed with construction, and the following spring the construction was completed.

We were shocked when the new Inspector from the Health Department condemned the construction before it could be occupied. It did not meet the new air-handling requirements, and until it did, no license to operate would be granted. The whole heating system had to be changed. New openings had to be made for air ducts to pass through concrete floors and walls. This added between thirty-five and forty thousand dollars, or about forty percent of the original cost of the whole wing to the total cost before we could use it.

CHAPTER XIV

MEDICAL INSURANCE

When I began my practice, hospital and medical insurance was hardly known. Patients and their families had always been responsible for paying their medical bills, and paying them was often a hardship, especially for poor families. For the poorest it was often impossible.

During the great depression of 1929-35, it was quite common for a doctor to be paid with goods and services rather than money, because many families had little monetary income. In rural areas family doctors were paid with farm produce, such as butter, eggs, chickens, vegetables, etc. Some families were too poor to even afford that, and in most such cases doctors generally provided their services without charge, or forgave substantial portions of their bills. People who were known indigents were essentially supported by various government entities under welfare programs. In rural areas the county governments and county welfare agencies would supply such things as food, clothing and shelter, but medical bills were largely ignored, or only small, token portions of them were approved and paid through the welfare agencies. However, I was never aware that anyone ever suffered severely or died for lack of medical care.

During the depression lack of funds kept many people from seeking medical advice until their illnesses were well advanced. This made making a correct diagnosis easier for the doctor, because it is much easier to make a diagnosis after the full-blown picture of the disease has developed, than it is when the first signs or symptoms appear.

During the great Depression interest in health and medical insurance grew slowly, and became increasingly greater during and immediately after World War II. Then doctors in Michigan, through their medical society, started a non-profit medical insurance company named Blue Cross, which covered doctor bills and certain other medical expenses. At about the same time hospital managements and administrators began a similar non-profit insurance company and named it Blue Shield. It covered hospital expenses. The purpose of both companies was to protect families from debt because of high medical expenses by having them regularly pay modest insurance premiums. Then if illness struck, there would be money available to pay both doctor and hospital bills. Patients were interested because it would, without great hardship, keep them from involuntarily going into debt. Doctors and hospitals were happy because the insurance made it much easier for them to collect money owed to them.

At first each non-profit company had its own organization, run by its own board of directors. The board for Blue Cross was made up of mostly doctors, and the board of Blue Shield was made up of mainly hospital people. Both of these corporations were successful, and did well for a number of years. Realizing that there was some duplication of operations between the two, especially in the record keeping, and thinking that operating cost savings might perhaps be passed on to their policy holders, the two companies merged, and combined both their governing boards and their operations. As one company they continued to serve their customers well.

From the beginning and as long as they were governed by boards of directors composed mainly of health care professionals, the insurance policies that Blue Cross and Blue Shield sold to the public were popular, and the system worked well. However, these early organizers made one crucial ***mistake.*** They sold ***service policies***, which promised ***payment without limit*** for illness, and the payment was to be made with the ***inherently limited funds*** available from policy premiums. In agreeing to owe and pay for medical services for policy holders, without putting price tags on them, they practically abolished competition for medical services, and removed the normal economic "brakes," which otherwise kept medical charges and costs in check. Insofar as medical expenses were concerned, ***their service policies made every policyholder a millionaire,*** and instilled into the medical consumer the "spare no expense" mind-set that is prevalent today. Although admirably humanitarian, these service policies were a formula for both the rapid escalation of prices and the proliferation of services. They are the root cause of the extreme increases in medical costs which we have experienced, and which we continue to experience. ***It would have been far better, and easier for both the insurance companies and their subscribers, if these doctors and hospital administrators had established only indemnity insurance policies, with definite fee schedules for covered illnesses, and left the financial relationship between doctor or hospital and patient undisturbed! It would then be left to the patient to decide how the indemnity sums allotted by the insurance policy should be spent,---- not the doctor,---- not the hospital!***

Unlike service policies ***indemnity policies*** do not take the consumer out of the payment system. They require his participation. Although it is possible to assign policy benefit payments in favor of the insured to third parties, those dollars, when paid, belong to the policy holder, and it is the policy holder who should have complete control over how they are spent. He must remain responsible for wisely choosing a policy to fit his needs. It must be large enough to cover the medical costs he incurs or is likely to incur. He must remain aware that he is responsible for paying the entire bill, including the amounts that fall above what his policy will pay. He can voluntarily reduce or eliminate such payments by buying a more expensive policy with higher payouts, but such a policy will cost more in premiums. With such choices to consider he is almost certain to have a greater interest in his own medical costs than does the patient of today, and he will be much more likely to reject unneeded, unnecessary or frivolous expenses, which, I am sorry to say, do exist in health care.

In practice an indemnity policy pays out the predetermined costs of the covered services received, but only up to the dollar amount limit specified in the policy for each service. Under this system insurance companies have a much easier time calculating the dollar premiums necessary for the various policies they offer. If the consumer is not satisfied with his coverage, the insurance company will find it relatively easy to raise the payout limits, and calculate the increase in premium needed to guarantee them. The consumer also has the option of lowering his health care premiums by lowering the policy payout dollar limits, and may instead choose to pay for an umbrella policy to cover any health care costs over and above those limits. ***Had Blue Cross/Blue Shield started in the beginning with indemnity policies, escalation of medical care costs would have been much more reasonable than they actually have been, because the patient would necessarily have been much more involved in "figuring the costs."***

Actually the original Blue Cross/Blue Shield programs worked well when its board consisted mostly of doctors and medical people. They worked so well that outside interests were soon attracted to them, and before the ordinary physician in Michigan became aware of what was going on, the large labor unions, particularly of the auto industry in Detroit, had taken over Blue Cross/Blue Shield, and its governing board. Shortly thereafter I was made aware of the fact that its governing board had increased in size to over fifty people,---- only three of which belonged to the medical field. From then on the cost of medical care escalated even more rapidly.

Other insurance companies also entered the medical insurance business, but mostly indemnified their policyholders. Policy payouts were set in certain specified dollar amounts for specified treatments and services. For me these companies were easier to deal with. There was generally less paperwork, and much less back and forth correspondence over payment amounts.

Blue Cross\Blue Shield on the other hand seemed always to be shaving amounts off of what I considered reasonable charges, and had some circuitous routes of payment, which did not make sense. Before long the "Blues" seemed to be at odds with many physicians in Michigan, and there were also many others, like me, who felt that it was not worth the time spent to argue with them about fees.

One Blue Cross/Blue Shield payment policy that did not make sense to me resulted in a sharp disagreement between us about the fees paid for minor surgery such as the removal of small tumors, excisional biopsies, and repair of accidental wounds. I could do such procedures in my office very well, but in order to do them, a surgical pack had to be prepared and sterilized ahead of time. I had to supply the surgical instruments, needles, suture materials, and surgical towels and drapes, and make sure that all was sterile when it came time to use them. Additionally I had to supply packets of sterile surgical gloves, skin preparation solutions, sterile vials of local anesthetic solutions, and postoperative dressings. We made up the packs, and sterilized them in an autoclave. We bought sutures in sterile packages and solutions in quart or gallon bottles. Blue Cross/Blue Shield refused to cover these expenses, which were necessary in order to do office surgery, yet they regularly **paid me the same surgical fee for a given procedure whether I did it in my office or in the hospital.** After I discovered this, the doctors of our clinic did all of their minor surgical procedures in the hospital across the street. We no longer prepared sterile packs for minor surgical procedures in the clinic, because Blue Cross\Blue Shield would not pay us for them, but they did pay the hospital.

Another dispute I had, this one with Blue Shield, was over the cost of hospital care. During the era when it was popular to complain that medical costs were rising too fast because there were too many hospital beds in existence, the Blues and the government agencies were clamoring for reductions in the length of hospital stays and the closing of hospital beds in order to reduce costs. Blue Shield told our hospital that its average hospital stay for treating **acute congestive heart failure** was far too long, and was therefore wasting money. At the time the average length of stay for this diagnosis had been reduced to about five days in Sparrow Hospital in Lansing, Michigan. Our average length of stay was still over ten days,---more than twice as long.

Acute Congestive Heart Failure is a serious emergency condition in which the heart muscle fails and does not have enough strength, for one reason or another, to propel the patient's blood adequately through his circulatory system. Blood backs up in the veins in the lungs, and fluid from it seeps into the air spaces, causing wheezing, coughing, shortness of breath and cyanosis. Lips often appear blue because the circulating blood is not adequately oxygenated and becomes dark. Sometimes blood backs up in the systemic (main body) circulation, and fluid leaks out into the tissues causing noticeable swelling, which is called edema.

Treatment is urgent and may be safely begun before any laboratory tests or x-rays are done. The main aim of initial treatment is to quickly take as much of the circulatory work-load away from the heart muscle as possible, reducing the amount of work it must do, by reducing both the patient's physical exertion and his mental anxiety to a minimum. Strict rest and small doses of morphine seem to help to accomplish this very well. We administer oxygen in order to saturate the red blood cells and the blood serum with it as fully as possible. We reduce the circulatory load by reducing the volume of blood that the heart must circulate. No, we do not bleed these people, as was done with favorable results in some cases of heart failure during the middle ages. We administer a diuretic drug instead, which stimulates the kidneys to remove fluid from the bloodstream much faster than normal. Finally, we administer Digitalis, which is an alkaloid drug, extracted from foxglove plants. When properly used, it slows the heart rate and seems to strengthen the heartbeat. This allows the heart to push a bigger volume of blood out into the circulation with each beat, and the heart therefore becomes more efficient.

When I started practice we had two forms of digitalis,---- powdered, dried digitalis leaf, which we put into capsules, and a liquid extract of digitalis leaves, which was administered by the drop. There was no practical way to test these substances to predetermine exactly how much digitalis alkaloid was present in any given batch, so digitalis was always administered relatively slowly and the results of its action carefully observed for signs of overdosage. Even the treatment we called "rapid digitalization" took about twelve hours to accomplish. Ordinarily it was not necessary to administer digitalis as rapidly as many people thought, because the patient's condition usually improved significantly as the early treatments mentioned previously took effect. The initial dose of digitalis given was usually between one-half and two-thirds of what we anticipated it would take to raise the digitalis alkaloid level in the patient's serum to the optimum treatment level. After the initial dose, smaller incremental doses were given every few hours while we watched the patient carefully for signs of digitalis toxicity or increasing heart failure. Several days were often needed to adjust the daily dose to a level that was ideal for the patient. There were not many things available to help us with this adjustment. We had to gradually increase the dose until observation of the patient showed signs of toxicity. We watched for nausea, irregularities in the heartbeat and subtle changes in the electrocardiogram. Once the patient had achieved a steady heartbeat, and a stable daily dose of digitalis had been found for him, we discharged him from the hospital.

In contrast to this old fashioned way of treating heart failure, Sparrow Hospital was using more modern technology. The active alkaloid drug in digitalis leaf had been isolated, and the pure drug, called digoxin, was available in pill form. Its strength was accurately known, and there was also a laboratory test available to measure its level in the blood serum. Rapid digitalization was now safer because, absent the variations in strength inherent in digitalis leaf or tincture preparations, a more exact calculated dose of digoxin could be given. It was much safer now to give the entire calculated dose at the beginning of treatment. Before any more was given the hospital laboratory could calculate the digoxin level in the patient's serum, and dosage adjustments could be monitored by repeating the test as needed. Frequent electrocardiograms, and later continuous cardiac monitoring were also used to follow the course of treatment. Thus it became possible for Sparrow Hospital to accomplish the same thing that we accomplished in our small hospital, and safely discharge the average case of congestive heart failure in five days. The only difference in the end result of these two situations, however, was that the stay in Sparrow Hospital had cost eight to ten times what it had cost to treat and discharge a patient who had exactly the same medical problem and attained exactly the same treatment result from the stay in our hospital!

As time went on Blue Cross\Blue Shield tried many things to try to contain costs. Most of them seemed to be aimed at reducing payments to doctors and hospitals. Equality and fairness were not always considered. Over a period of time discrepancies gradually appeared in their physician payment schedules. Some doctors were paid more than others for identical procedures, presumably because of the location of their offices. Instead of setting fees paid to physicians according to the service rendered, Blue Cross set up physician fee profiles, by keeping track of all of the charges that each individual physician made. The list of these charges created a "profile" of charges for each physician. Then the profile was scrutinized, and if the doctor had reduced his charge for any reason to any patient for any procedure, Blue Cross established the lower charge for that procedure as the standard charge in the doctor's profile, and it became the new figure to be used in calculating future payments. Worse yet, when a young physician entered practice, he had no fee profile, and could charge much more for his services by setting his initial fees extraordinarily high at the very beginning. Then as his profile was established it reflected these higher fees, and they became the standard payments that he received. It actually happened in my family that my brother, a surgeon who trained for his surgical career at the Mayo Clinic in Rochester, Minnesota, was receiving a fee of $650 for doing a cholecystectomy (removal of a gall bladder), when his son, who had also trained at the Mayo Clinic, started his practice and was paid almost twice as much for exactly the same operation. With such things happening it did not take long for doctors to try to increase and protect their profiles by maintaining unrealistically high billings for their services in order to always be charging higher fees than the insurance companies allowed.

I remember that I submitted a bill to Blue Cross for $35 for removal of a large area of perianal venereal warts, a procedure which took about half an hour When their check came, they paid something like

$4.50. I sent my objection to them by mail, and eventually received a letter in return stating that only one lesion had been removed, and that was their allowance for each lesion. I sent in a second bill for "Removal of more than 450,000 lesions at $4.50 per lesion, together with a letter from a Lansing dermatologist who stated that an aggregation of *condyloma accuminata,* of the size which had been removed, contained at least 450,000 individual warts. As a result Blue Cross sent me $30.50, the difference between what I had billed in the beginning and what they had already paid. The argument had cost me more in time and money than I had made by caring for the patient.

Blue Cross allowed doctors to participate in several ways. One was to be a Blue Cross participant, always accept what was allowed in the fee schedule and agree to not charge the patient any more than that. This was great for the insurance company because they could assure their enrollees full coverage for all doctor bills with no extra charges as long as they went to a participating doctor. In another arrangement Blue cross paid the doctor according to their payment schedule and allowed the doctor to bill the patient for the difference. This was not as good for the doctor as it sounds, because many patients ignored the extra charges, and it was expensive to send out bills. Often the amount owed was small enough that sending a bill and collecting it would cost the physician more than he could receive. However, if the physician failed to bill each patient for the extra amount, and Blue Cross found out about it, they reduced that physician's allowed profile fee accordingly.

Our most colossal mistreatment by Blue Cross happened at about the time I retired from practice. The Eaton Rapids Medical Clinic, of which I had been a founder and was a practicing member, had added a licensed psychologist to its staff. He was hired with the approval of Blue Cross, and had been working in the Clinic for over two years, when Blue Cross sent out a couple of people to inspect his records. He wrote his reports into the single clinic record, which was kept by the clinic for each patient. The result of this inspection was a letter from Blue Cross, which rejected some $40,000.00 of our psychologist's billings which had been submitted since the he had started to work at the clinic, and stated further that it was withholding all sums payable to our clinic until all of this money had been paid back!!!

Medicare and Medicaid seem to have adopted the philosophy of service policies from Blue Cross/Blue Shield, which I believe has added drastically to medical costs in the United States. Of the two, Medicaid is the most onerous, and I shall tell about it first.

Medicaid was and is intended to care for the indigent, and services that are free to them should be simply and correctly called ***welfare.*** Although nobody seems to be calling it that, that is exactly what it is. In the beginning it was intended that Medicaid pay for medical care for the truly needy. Today, however, it also picks up the tab for mentally, morally and socially bankrupt people, as well as a horde of lazy ones, who are most certainly citizen liabilities in our society. Scrutinized in any light, this is still ***welfare***, and nothing else.

While I was in practice, both doctors and hospitals would, year after year, be informed early in each year that Medicaid would pay during that year a certain percent of their usual charges for treatment of Medicaid patients. The rate was often set between 50 and 70 percent of usual charges, and at those levels it usually meant no take home pay from the treatment of Medicaid patients for the doctor, and an actual loss to the hospitals for caring for them in the hospital. Then later in the year, often as early as October, Medicare would announce that its funds for the year were exhausted, and there would be no more payments to either doctors or hospitals for the rest of the year. I believe that this, perhaps with some variation, is still going on today. In any case it is safe to say that doctors make at best no profit from Medicaid patients, and hospitals sustain sizeable losses from them.

But isn't what Medicaid recipients receive from doctors and hospitals actually ***welfare?*** Of course it is! Just as what they receive from the government in food stamps, clothing and shelter is welfare, what they receive free from doctors, and what they receive free of charge from hospitals is also welfare.

This gives rise to the next question. ***If doctors and hospitals are handing out so much WELFARE, how can they stay in business?*** The answer is simple. Doctors make their living from their other patients, and make enough more from their other patients to offset their losses incurred because they have treated Medicaid patients, and hospitals collect enough more from their other patients to cover the losses sustained by them from caring for Medicaid patients. Were it not so, hospitals would be very quickly forced to go out of business, and many physicians would quit practice.

Nowhere is this easier to demonstrate with numbers than it is in the business of nursing homes with skilled nursing care and rehabilitation services. My friends in the business tell me that nationwide over 70% of the patients in these facilities are paid for by Medicaid. The cost for privately paying patients in these nursing homes averages about $60,000.00 per year (now in the year 2002), while Medicaid payments average a few dollars above $100.00 per day for each patient, or approximately $40,000.00 per year. The difference, about $20,000.00 per year, is what each private pay patient contributes to make up the deficit created by Medicaid patients in these nursing homes.

Now consider that welfare is the responsibility of the government, and the government is the responsibility of all of the people in the country. Are not the dollars which the doctors and hospitals are giving to Medicaid patients the equivalent of taxes paid to the government? I certainly think so. Because both doctors and hospitals must include, in their collections from other patients, enough money to cover their Medicare deficits in order to stay in business, the ultimate payers of these "taxes" are the patients who pay their bills by other means. To say it another way, the private pay patients are selectively chosen to pay for the deficits caused by Medicaid. Their money goes to pay the costs of welfare that is really the responsibility of the government of all of the people. The rest of the populace does not contribute. Therefore this process appears to be blatantly unfair taxation. It is selective taxation of those individual citizens who, directly or indirectly, pay regular hospital bills and/or doctor bills. Going one step further, we might even consider doctors and hospitals to be the tax collection agencies working for the government without pay.

Medicare - Because I am a senior citizen and enrolled in Medicare, I now am quite familiar with it, and with many of the supplemental insurance policies to Medicare that exist. I have no quarrel with Medicare, except that it has expanded its benefits too much without collecting an equivalent amount in insurance premiums. Medicare charges a large, deductible "admission fee" for patients who are admitted to the hospital, and after that it pays most of the rest of the hospital costs of the admission. It also pays 80% of specifically approved charges for specific outpatient services. The other 20% is a deductible, but Medicare recipients can buy Medicare supplemental insurance to pay both the hospital admission fee and the 20% deductibles. Medicare Part B covers the outpatient services, and for this coverage Medicare charged me a $600 insurance premium last year. This premium is much too small for the coverage promised. This same year my premium payment for a good commercial Medicare Supplement Insurance policy, which I buy to cover the Medicare deductible amounts, was over eight times that much.

Medicare differs financially from Medicaid in that one may depend upon it, and it has through the years come to some agreement with the hospitals on hospital costs and reimbursements. It has abandoned some of the characteristics of full service insurance policies. It has set definite fee schedules for doctors, which apply uniformly to all services, and the 80% payment that Medicare makes is for practical purposes guaranteed. Medicare's arrangement with hospitals is much more complicated, and requires inspection and auditing of hospital books, but under the present system it should be possible for a well run hospital to break even insofar as the care of Medicare patients is concerned. It has also placed the responsibility for billing for services to Medicare patients upon the doctor, and this has brought about a high degree of standardization of the process, which saves a huge amount of misunderstood, frustrating interaction between Medicare, the doctor and the patient. Many doctors in our area find it easier and more profitable to also submit their billings to the companies that supply supplemental insurance to Medicare, and this also has made things easier for their patients.

The relationship between Medicare and certain doctors remains strained because Medicare has placed caps on the cost of many services and procedures, drastically reducing and sometimes eliminating profits from them. In some cases the overhead cost of doing certain surgical operations is more than Medicare allows for the procedure. It is not yet a perfect system.

CHAPTER XV

EATON RAPIDS MEDICAL CLINIC

There were four doctors in the Stimson Medical Group, when construction began on the new Eaton Rapids Community Hospital. Dr. Eber B. Sherman, M.D. had joined us immediately after he completed his tour of military service. The prospect of continuing our office practices in the old hospital building after the Stimson Hospital ceased to exist was not heartening, and after discussing the coming situation, we decided to build a new office building, and to build it as near to the new hospital as possible. Fortunately we were able to buy land across Spicerville Road from the hospital site, on the same side of Highway M-99. It was the only land belonging to the Wallace Swank Farm that was West of Highway M-50, and Wallace agreed to sell it to us. Once again I drew floor plans, which were based upon the examining rooms I had seen at the Mayo Clinic. There were four physician offices, ten examining rooms, a laboratory and pharmacy area, a reception counter, a business office, and, at the front of the building, a large, cheerful waiting room with a fieldstone fireplace and big windows. We also decided to change the name of our medical group to EATON RAPIDS MEDICAL CLINIC, the change to become effective when we moved into our new building.

The four of us, Dr. Bert VanArk, Dr Herman VanArk, Dr. Sherman and I, formed a second partnership for the purpose of owning and managing the new office building. In the beginning we each contributed equal lump sums of money to it, and were then able to arrange financing with a mortgage from our local bank. When in operation the Medical Clinic paid rent to the new Building Partnership. This money in turn was used to make the mortgage payments, pay taxes and other expenses. We engaged Professional Management of Battle Creek, Michigan, the firm that had helped me in starting my practice, to oversee and audit the books of both partnerships.

One day, when the new medical clinic building was nearing completion, a new doctor who was looking for a place to start his medical practice, happened to arrive in town on Kinneyville Road, which, as it joined Highway M-99, ran almost into the doorstep of the new hospital. He was Owen S. (Stuart) Erhard, M.D., a graduate of the Seventh Day Adventist Medical School in Loma Linda, California. He stopped to inquire, and was directed to our offices in the Stimson Hospital Building.

He did many of the things that I had done when I decided to settle in Eaton Rapids, and after a few days he accepted our offer to become a member of our group and a new member of the EATON RAPIDS MEDICAL CLINIC when it started up. He became the fifth doctor to join our medical group, and he practiced with us for a long time. His wife, Beaty, delivered several children, and had some minor surgery done in our hospital. Eventually, the Erhard family left our area for California, where Dr. Erhard entered a residency and eventually became a board certified anesthesiologist, and continued his practice of anesthesia in California.

Dr. Vernon Butler, M.D., also a graduate of the Seventh Day Adventist School, also soon joined the group, but he did not stay long. It is my impression that he did not like the work of general practice, but I don't exactly remember why he left.

The property we had acquired from Wallace Swank was a triangular piece with frontage on both roads. Before we could arrange the financing for our building we had to clear our title to it. The Marathon Oil Company owned the drilling rights to the Swank Farm, and the bank, which was to provide the money for our construction costs considered this to be a significant blemish on the title. Richard Robinson, who practiced law in Eaton Rapids before he became a judge, represented us, and arranged to have Marathon Oil Company remove their drilling claim on that part of the Swank property that we now owned. In order to save time we had Dick Robinson prepare the necessary papers and drive with me to the Marathon Oil Company headquarters in Ohio. This took only one day. We met with two company lawyers for half an hour, then finished up the signing, and were on our way back home. I was so impressed with the friendly but business-like treatment that we received at the Marathon offices, that I have ever since bought gasoline at Marathon Service Stations whenever possible.

We did hire an architect for our building project, and after the clinic building was finished, I, for one, was sorry that we had done so. Some of the specifications that accompanied his plans made no sense to me, but as I pointed out the mistakes I thought he was making, he acted like a prima donna, and would not listen. First I pointed out that the ceiling insulation was too thin. He wouldn't listen. Specified in the plans were a gas furnace to heat the building, which put out only 140,000 BTU of heat per hour, and a hot water heater with an output of 320,000 BTU per hour to supply hot water to 14 lavatory sinks. I pointed out, to no avail, that these numbers seemed to be reversed. During our first winter in practice in that building it was too cold in the examining rooms to examine patients unless we also had portable electric heaters operating in them. We asked him to correct the problem, but he denied responsibility. We sued in court and won. As a result we received enough money to replace the undersized furnace, and kept the oversized hot water heater in operation. The air conditioning unit he had specified for the building was a ten-ton unit, which was large enough, but it kept breaking down, and we were frequently waiting for parts from the manufacturer needed to repair it.

Another problem was the matter of sewage disposal. Our property was just outside the city limits, and there were no sewer lines to hook up to. We needed a septic tank and drain field, and the county health department required that the drain field contain 3,000 feet of properly buried drain tile. This was much, much more than was needed, but our arguments went unheeded, and we planted the 3,000 feet of septic drainage tile under the lawn to the West of the parking lot. Ironically, the city extended the sewer line about two years later, and the clinic was able to hook up to it.

When we moved into the new building, we engaged Mrs. Effie Fuller to be the overall manager of our business, and she was a winner, who excelled not only at managing the business but also at handling people.

With Dr Erhard working in the Clinic, the need for more office space soon became apparent, so we borrowed more money and doubled the number of offices and examining rooms. This time we installed three home type furnaces with air conditioners to service the new area. This arrangement worked so well that when the main heating or air conditioning broke down, we could keep the whole building at a reasonable temperature with only those three furnaces operating until repairs could be made.

The highlight adventure of this new building project came during the time when the basement was being dug. Almost exactly in the center of what was to be the new basement, a huge rock was uncovered. It was larger than an automobile, and much too big for the digging equipment to get it out of the excavation, so the decision was made to use dynamite to break it up so it could be removed in pieces.

About the middle of the next morning I was operating in the hospital surgery. Dr Sherman was the anesthetist, and I believe that Dr Erhard was assisting. From the direction of the Clinic across the street came a loud explosion, and instantly we all knew that the rock had been dynamited. However, when we arrived at the Clinic at about noon, we learned that the rock had not been broken at all, although the explosion had blown in all of the windows at the rear of the clinic building. Most of the examining rooms were located across the back of the building, and were immediately peppered inside with shattered glass. The big rock was still there, lying intact, in the basement excavation.

Our office manager, Effie Fuller, quickly sized up the situation. She went across the highway to the supermarket and bought a number of brooms and dustpans. Every available person was recruited to sweep up glass. She also had someone come in with some plastic sheeting and cover the glassless window frames. Heat in the rooms was no problem because it was early summer. We were able to begin office hours at 1:00 p.m. as if nothing had happened.

We were told that the dynamiting had not been successful because the people doing it had not been well trained. They had placed the dynamite on top of the rock, and the explosion there had not damaged it at all. The next day another crew came in to do the job. They placed the explosives correctly, and shattered the rock without any further damage to the building.

Next to join the Eaton Rapids Medical Clinic staff was Dr. Vernon Butler, M.D. He was also a graduate of the Seventh Day Adventist Medical School in Loma Linda, California. He was well trained and a capable doctor, but apparently did not like the life and the practice in Eaton Rapids, and after only a short time, left to work elsewhere.

Soon to join the Clinic was Dr. Beth Yankee, who came to us from the church mission field in Nigeria, Africa, where she had had extensive medical experience, from major surgery to handling infectious epidemics. She had done several hundred Caesarian Sections, and had taught Nigerian natives how to do a number of surgical operations, particularly the repair of inguinal hernias. Before her term of missionary work was finished she had served as the director of a large mission hospital, and in that position had experienced a huge epidemic of Bubonic Plague among the natives. Her parents lived in Manistee, Michigan and her father was a minister. Beth was not only a good doctor, but also handled patients well. While she was in Eaton Rapids she married Andy Jensen, and soon they moved to Arizona where she finished out her medical career, and is now retired.

Dr. Susan Courtnage Stipanuk and Dr. Gerald Stipanuk, husband and wife, were internal medicine specialists who came to us together from residency programs in Lansing. Susan gave birth to two children in our hospital, but the marriage didn't last. Gerald left to hold a number of different medical positions in the surrounding areas, but Dr. Susan Courtnage remained, and is still living and practicing in Eaton Rapids.

Dr. Howard Luckenbill, D.O. came to us from an internship at Lansing General Hospital (Osteopathic), and we found him to be a good doctor too. He did not stay very long, but left to go into a residency in anesthesia somewhere in the Eastern U.S. I have lost track of him.

Dr. Barbara Supanich also was with the Clinic for a few years. She was a Catholic Nun with a medical degree, and she still belonged to her Catholic Order. I recall that her paychecks went to the Order, and she was given a small allowance upon which to live. When she left Eaton Rapids it was to practice in a small town in Northern Lower Michigan, where she stayed for an extended period. Now she trains family practice residents at Munson Medical Center in Traverse City, Michigan. My wife still speaks of her as "Sister Doctor Barbara."

Dr. Courtnage's father, a surgeon nearing retirement, also joined the Clinic for a short time before he actually did retire.

My two sons, Dr. Albert H. Meinke, III, M.D. and Dr. William B. Meinke, M.D. each spent several years with the Clinic before they moved on with their careers.

For a short time we also had a pediatrician in the group, a woman who was just out of her residency program. I don't remember her name. She could not stay long because she was unable to cover even her overhead expenses by the amount of work that she did.

Of the four original members of the Eaton Rapids Medical Clinic, Dr. Herman VanArk died suddenly while riding upon a tractor mower and mowing his lawn. At the time he was still in practice. Dr. Bert VanArk died before he retired completely. Dr. Eber Sherman has retired and lives with his wife on Lake Louise in Northern Lower Michigan, and I retired in 1984, and ever since have lived with my wife on the shore of Torch Lake in Antrim County, Michigan.

Eaton Rapids Medical Clinic came to an end when those of the group who owned the building sold all of their interest in the real estate to The Eaton Rapids Community Hospital, and it is now a part of Eaton Rapids Medical Center.

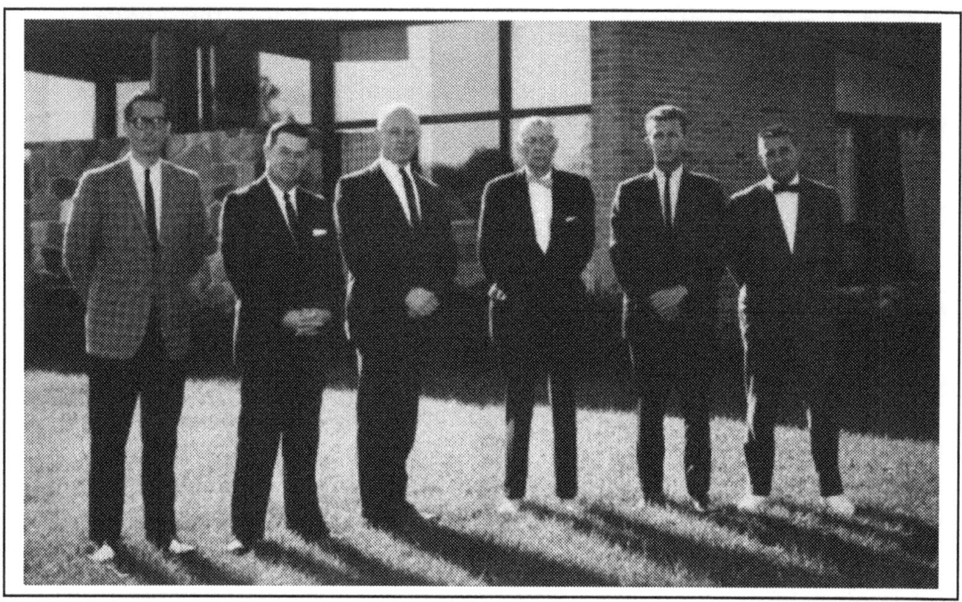

Pictured here are the six physicians who practiced in the new medical partnership, THE EATON RAPIDS MEDICAL CLINIC. They are: (left to right) O.S. "Stu" Erhard, M.D., Herman F. VanArk, M.D., Albert H. Meinke, Jr., M.D., Bert VanArk, M.D., Vernon Butler, M.D., and Eber B. Sherman, M.D.

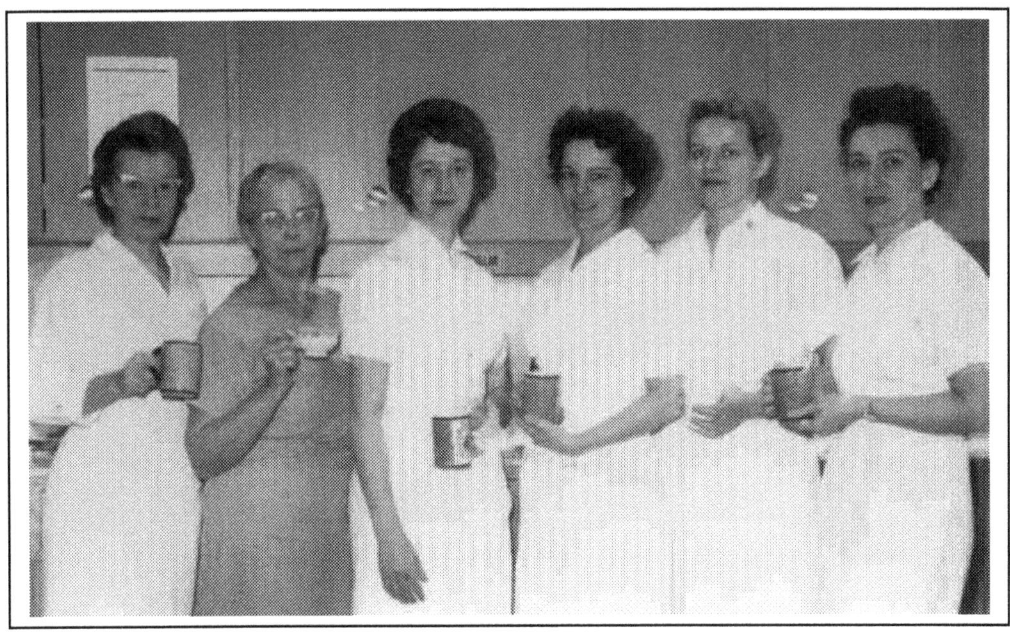

Nurses and office assistants who worked at the EATON RAPIDS MEDICAL CLINIC when it first began. Shown here (from left to right) are Mary VanAuker, Bernice Bowman, Sharon Leatherberry (married name Garnant), RosemaryTaylor, R.N., Eileen Vance, R.N. (married name Hawblitzel), and Elizabeth "Betty" Card, R.N. Bernice Bowman received her medical training at the Harriet Chapman School of Nursing in Eaton Rapids, and was not only a nurse, but also a surgical technician.

CHAPTER XVI

OBSTETRIC SERVICES

In very early days most babies were born at home, but after the Harriet Chapman Hospital opened in Eaton Rapids in 1918, it soon became customary for babies to be born there, or in a maternity home which was located nearby. The maternity home had closed by the time I arrived in town, and the hospital's name had been changed to Stimson Hospital. Almost all babies in the area were born there, except occasionally, when, by accident, one was born too quickly for the mother to get to the hospital.

All of the doctors in the Stimson Medical Group included obstetrics in their practices. Later after the group became the Eaton Rapids Medical Clinic, and Dr. Beth Yankee was included in the staff, all six physicians regularly delivered babies. There seemed to be an abundant number of obstetric cases, and I believed it was because not only were fathers invited into the delivery room, but also our services were also substantially less expensive than they were in the larger hospitals.

After a few years of smooth operation, the State Health Department inspected and condemned the obstetrical areas in our relatively new hospital. Ignoring the excellent morbidity and mortality records that our Obstetrics Unit was turning in each year, they cited, among other things, the fact that the location of our newborn nursery was across the main hall of the hospital from the delivery room. This made it necessary to carry the babies through the "contaminated" hall when they left the delivery room, and whenever they were taken out of the nursery to their mothers for feeding. Nothing we suggested would satisfy these "powers that be" except to build a new wing, exclusively for obstetrics, which could be adequately closed off from the rest of the hospital. Obstetrics was such an important part of our medical care then, that the hospital, extended itself financially, and added the new obstetrical wing to the hospital building. This action was taken solely because this threat of condemnation and closure was hanging over our heads.

The building project was itself not without its own problems, and in the chapter on Regulator Problems I have outlined the hard time and expense that the Health Department created for us by first approving the construction plans, then disapproving the building before it could be used.

After the extensive alterations to the new wing were completed and approved we were allowed to use it. Obstetrics in the new unit went very well for a few years, but one day our hospital was notified that we would receive an official visit from the head of the Michigan Department of Public Health. I have forgotten this physician's name, but I distinctly remember that I had a bad feeling about his impending visit, and was certain that no good would come of it. Being medical director of the hospital, I was present at the meeting, which was held in the basement of the hospital using the library as a conference room. Everyone attending was seated around the large conference table, with Dr. "Big Shot" at the head.

Our visitor explained that he had been in the private practice of obstetrics and gynecology, but had dropped out of it to become head of the state health department. I wondered why, and suspected that he had quit the practice because he found that he couldn't make a living at it. After the preliminary introductions were over, it did not take him long to tell us that he had come to convince us to shut down our obstetrics department and stop delivering babies in Eaton Rapids, because it was not safe.

His statement shocked me. I knew all about the records we kept. We hardly ever had a fetal death to report, and never any that could be blamed upon poor treatment. We had had absolutely no maternal deaths either. For a time I argued back and forth with Dr. Big Shot, and during the exchange he stated several times that it was dangerous for a mother to be delivered in any hospital, which had less than 100 births per year. I couldn't believe that, and had to disagree completely. Normally we had well over 100 deliveries per year, but the previous year had been unusually slow for us, and we had had only 98. This was below the magic 100 number for the first time since I had come to town. We always kept track of the annual number of births, and our biggest year had seen almost 300 deliveries.

Our discussion continued at some length, during which I got the impression that our visiting doctor had flaunted his Ob-Gyn Specialty around in the Health Department offices, and that the arguments he was presenting to us were his ideas that he was passing on to us as the policies of the Health Department. The longer we talked the more ridiculous some of his statements became, until finally he stated emphatically and with a vigorous wave of his arm,

"I WILL SHUT DOWN YOUR MATERNITY DEPARTMENT!!"

I answered promptly,

"You will not! Not without a fight!"

After the meeting had ended, and I had time to think about what had happened, there were several things that seemed peculiar. This doctor had come to ask us the close our obstetrical department. To me that meant that he knew he could not legally do it without our voluntary cooperation. He had been ill prepared, and had presented nothing to back up his claims that obstetrics in small hospitals was dangerous. I knew that the State

Health Department had a computer, and I wondered why it wasn't being used to gather this kind of information. I was so sure that his statement, that small hospitals' obstetrical care was dangerous, was wrong, that I had to prove it was false.

To begin I decided to review all of our hospital charts of births from the time I arrived in town up to the current year. Fortunately when we had moved the Stimson Hospital equipment to the new hospital, we also moved the old hospital records, and they had all been kept. Between the records of the two hospitals more than 25 years of obstetrical history in Eaton Rapids were available to me. I reviewed charts for several months, and logged statistics. This work was done at night in the medical records room, and when I was finished I was pleased to find that the averages, for all of those years in every statistical category, demonstrated that our hospital's obstetrical care had been substantially better than the state averages for the several most recent years reported. Our hospital had certainly not been a dangerous place in which to have a baby!

Another thing I learned incidentally from my survey was that there had been over 6,000 babies born during that time (6,033 I believe), and well over half of them had been my cases.

The numbers I had uncovered began to interest me, and I decided to investigate even more. I requested the State fetal and maternal statistics from the health department for the latest five years for which they were available, and the Department obliged. I had always felt that health statistics numbers fed to the public were presented in an underhanded manner. Perinatal deaths, which are deaths inside the uterus after twenty weeks of gestation up to a newborn baby's age of one week, were stated in deaths per 1,000 live births. The public was accustomed to thinking in terms of percentages, and I believe often misinterpreted the number as deaths per 100 births. I wondered if the public was being misled in other ways.

With this new information spread out before me, the next numbers that caught my eye were the maternal deaths for that five-year period. There were five recorded maternal deaths in the State of Michigan during that time. Two of them had been assigned to the same hospital, the Osteopathic Hospital in Traverse City, and another was stated to have happened in Eaton County.

There were only two hospitals in Eaton County,---- ours and Hayes-Green-Beach Hospital in Charlotte. I knew that there had been no maternal deaths ever in our hospital, so I phoned the administrator at Hayes-Green-Beach, and asked her to tell me about the maternal death that they had had there.

"We haven't had any maternal deaths," she stated. "Where did you get that information?"

I assured her that there was a maternal death attributed to Eaton County in the State Vital Statistics, and since neither hospital knew anything about it, I would investigate some more. Eventually I learned that the case being reported was that of a Hispanic woman who had come to Eaton County with her family to work in the farm harvests, and who had had some prenatal examinations under the supervision of the Health Department while she was in Eaton County. The family then went back to Texas, and she had died there several months later. I never learned the cause. Was this an official Michigan maternal death, the fault of the hospital and medical professions in Michigan? I THINK NOT!!!!!!!

When I contacted the osteopathic hospital in Traverse City, the administration cooperated fully, and sent me copies of the cover sheets containing the summary of the hospital admissions in both of the maternal death cases. The first one was of a woman who was six months along in her pregnancy when she died as the result of an automobile accident. The prematurely born baby didn't survive either, so this was listed as both a maternal and a fetal death. HOW ABSURD!!!!!!! The second case involved a death, due to excessive bleeding during and after labor. From the information available I doubted that this patient could have been saved, but I did believe that, because no other disease condition had been diagnosed, it may have been properly labeled as a maternal death. The other two listed maternal deaths, did have obstetric diagnoses, and were probably also legitimate maternal deaths. Actually there had been three maternal deaths in all of Michigan during that five-year period, and considering the number of successful births during that same time, this is certainly not a very high mortality rate.

In order to get some more accurate statistics on births in hospitals delivering less than 100 babies per year, I sent a letter to the administrator of all thirty such hospitals in Michigan, asking for the same five years of their obstetrical statistics, and I received prompt replies from about 80% of them. In general their track records were about as good as ours, and all but one or two of the records were better than the state averages.

Some time later the State Health Department came out with some statistics of its own, which listed the perinatal and neonatal deaths for hospitals divided into five groups, according to the number of births they had each year. ***After these numbers became known, we heard nothing more about how dangerous obstetrics was in small hospitals***. The five groups were:

Hospitals with less than 100 deliveries annually
Hospitals with 100 to 500 deliveries annually
Hospitals with 501 to 1500 deliveries annually
Hospitals with 1501 to 2500 deliveries annually
Hospitals with over 2500 deliveries annually

A sixth category was also included which contained the statistics of the Obstetrical Department of the University of Michigan Hospital, which were better than those of any of the groups listed. The hospitals with up to 100 births per year had the best perinatal and neonatal records. Next best was the group with up to 500 births per year. Then as the size of the group increased the record became poorer, until the level of the University Hospital was reached, and there it suddenly was the best record of all of the groups.

A State Senate Hearing to take up the question of changes in the laws regarding obstetrical practice was advertised soon after these State Health Department numbers became available. I applied to speak at the hearing, and was granted permission. Before going I prepared the childbirth statistics from my own survey of small hospitals for presentation, and had them in written form to give to the senators. I also prepared a table with the Department of Public Health statistics, which clearly demonstrated that as hospitals got larger their perinatal statistics got worse, but when the level of obstetric expertise at the University of Michigan Hospital was reached, the perinatal mortality numbers were sharply reduced to levels below those of all of the other groups. I told the senators that I believed that these statistics were true, and that any good general practitioner who delivered babies in a small town could have told them, before the survey, what the findings would be, and why.

The small town doctor is no dummy. His patients are his friends. He has the ability to anticipate obstetrical complications well ahead of time, and refer those patients who are likely to have major trouble to specialists. Where? In the cities! These specialists practice in the larger hospitals. These larger hospitals receive the higher risk cases referred to them from the out of town practitioners using the smaller hospitals. A local physician is normally not comfortable in taking care of exceptionally obese mothers, mothers with toxemia of pregnancy, mothers with diabetes, mothers with hypertension or kidney disease, mothers with blood clotting problems, etc. All over the United States the bulk of the high-risk obstetric cases end up in the larger hospitals, and because of this their higher perinatal mortality records are neither surprising, nor are they out of line. As for the University Hospital, its record was the only one not skewed, as were the others, by calamities which begin away from the hospital, i.e. unanticipated fetal deaths in which the fetus is already dead inside the uterus before the mother's arrival at the hospital, or, through no fault of the doctor or hospital, the fetus could not be saved. Patients at the University Hospital were referred by doctors from all over the state, and very rarely arrived in a state of extreme emergency or with the fetus already in a moribund condition, as they do at all other hospitals. Such cases are not likely to be thrust, unanticipated, upon the University Hospital as they are upon the rest of the hospitals. But such cases add to hospital mortality numbers, and I suspect that if we were to remove all such cases from every hospital's perinatal mortality record, many of them would match the University Hospital's mortality rates.

To illustrate the kinds of obstetric cases that are not presented to the University Hospital I shall describe several cases from my own practice, which added to my hospital's perinatal mortality rate.

One that I recall clearly was the case of one of my patients who arrived at the hospital with the baby's body already out of the vagina and the head stuck inside, and by the time she arrived at the hospital the baby had already died of suffocation. I had examined her in the office less than a week earlier, and everything was fine. The baby's head was down in a normal cephalic (head) presentation, but, since then, the baby's position had changed into a breech presentation. Then labor had begun, and was so powerful that the baby's body was born well before the patient could arrive at the hospital. This perinatal death was included in the statistics of our hospital.

Another case that I vividly recall was that of a mother carrying twins, who went into labor at about six and one half months of gestation and began suddenly to bleed very heavily. When I examined her in the Emergency Room, I found the cervix partly dilated with a placenta (afterbirth) presenting itself in the opening. I was able to reduce the blood loss immediately by setting up a tamponade with surgical packs placed into the vagina, but labor continued, and I knew that as the cervix continued to dilate, more and more of the placenta would separate and the bleeding would worsen. I could still hear both fetal heartbeats. The babies were far along enough so that there was a chance that they would survive if they were delivered immediately. If the labor and the bleeding were allowed to continue, their chances of survival were about zero, and the mother's survival was in doubt. I delivered the babies by emergency caesarian section, and except for being premature and small, they were both alive and appeared to be in good condition. As soon as the placenta was delivered, the mother returned to a normal post partum state with only a moderate anemia from the blood loss to show for her ordeal. Subsequently she made a good, full recovery, but her babies proved to be too premature and only survived a few days. They represented two more perinatal deaths in our hospital's statistics.

Another case was that of a woman who's due date had arrived. All of her prenatal examinations had been normal. I had examined her in my office less than a week before, and everything was fine. She arrived at the hospital in labor, and when I examined her there, the labor appeared to be progressing normally, but I could not hear the baby's heart beat. After listening for it for a long time, I was sure that the baby was dead. When the baby was born some hours later, it was truly dead, and the cause of death was quite obvious. There was a tightly tied knot in the umbilical cord near its attachment to the placenta. The cord was unusually long and was also wrapped twice around one of the baby's ankles. The baby's kicking had tightened the knot, and the baby died before birth, and probably even before the labor began, from lack of oxygen.

In Michigan the law regarding stillbirths was specific. A woman, who is over half way through a pregnancy (20 weeks or more), who aborts (miscarries), is presumed to have delivered a stillborn child. The birth and death had to be recorded. Years ago both a birth certificate and a death certificate had to be filled out. More recently a certificate of stillbirth, which reports both the birth and the death in one document, is being used, but the consequences remain the same. Cases like these, and those previously described, generally don't reach the University Hospital, and, I repeat, if such deaths were to be removed from the records of out-state hospitals, I speculate that their records would be about equal to those of the University Hospital.

The materials, which the Health Department had sent to me, also included the death certificate diagnoses of all of the perinatal deaths in the state in each of those five years. They interested me greatly, and I picked out one of the years in the early 1970's to study these diagnoses with the idea in mind of determining how many of these babies might have been saved. What I found was surprising. Out of almost 300 deaths, I found only 12 that I thought might possibly have been prevented. Most of the rest had horrible anomalies, malformations and deformations that had no chance for sustained life, or such a degree of prematurity that survival was not possible. The perinatal death rate for those five years was about 12 per thousand live births per year. If only the babies that I thought might have survived, with perhaps some different treatment than they had received, had been listed separately as possibly preventable deaths, it would come to only a fraction of one death per thousand live births per year. But this was not a figure that the politicians were passing out to the public. Figures like that were not likely to improve the possibilities of getting more funding for their bureaucracies. As reported, the number of perinatal deaths in the State now remains around 10 per thousand live births per year, almost all of which I truly believe cannot be prevented by any means presently known.

This realization prompted me to look at the perinatal death numbers for as many years past as possible, and again I was surprised. Before antibiotics were available, before we knew how to prevent and treat the problems of Rh blood type incompatibility, before we had neonatologists, and before we had thrown massive numbers of dollars at many perceived obstetrical problems, the perinatal death rates in the years during the 1930's were 14 to 15 deaths per 100,000 births each year. In the

1970's it had improved to about 12 per 100,000. Today I believe that the number stands around 10. This is improvement, but it may not be due to our efforts at improving medical practice. It could be that because of increased knowledge and use of birth control, fewer horrible freaks are being born than there were in the 1930's.

Although the Health Department failed to close down our obstetrics service, our Obstetrics Department eventually died for lack of physician support. By the time I retired in 1984 Dr. Bert VanArk and Dr. Herman VanArk were gone. Dr. Erhard had left for California, and Dr. Beth Yankee would soon leave for Arizona. The physicians who remained to use the hospital were not very interested in obstetrics, so Eaton Rapids Community Hospital was eventually compelled, for financial reasons, to close out its Obstetrics Department.

CHAPTER XVII

ANESTHESIA

During my years in Eaton Rapids the administration of anesthetics changed dramatically. The changes occurred gradually, but made giant leaps in safety and efficiency when anesthesia machines came into use, and again when endotracheal intubation became practical. As changes in anesthesia practices evolved, so did surgical procedures. Operations, which were once most difficult to do under the older methods of anesthesia, became much easier, and operative procedures which were once considered very risky, were made not only possible, but were proved to be quite safe as well. Anesthesia was particularly important to me because surgery was the part of medical practice that I liked most, and the marked improvement in anesthesia practices made possible many of the surgical procedures that I later did.

It was a well-established principle in any surgical procedure, that the surgeon was always the captain of the ship. He was not only in charge of everything, but was legally responsible for all that was done by others assisting in the operation. This meant that whenever I operated, I was responsible for everything that anyone else in the operating room did. The group of people involved there usually consisted of the assistant surgeon, the anesthetist, the scrub nurse, the circulating nurse, and anyone else who was called into the operating room to participate in any treatment of the patient. Because this principle had been upheld in the courts and had well established legal standing, I took it very seriously, and paid close attention to details in the operating room.

The patient's position on the operating table was important, because awkward positioning and pressure upon particular areas of the body have been known to cause more or less permanent nerve damage and paralysis. Another worry arose whenever we applied external heat to keep the patient warm and prevent lowering of the body temperature. I was always insistent that hot water bottles be not too hot.

In the early years my greatest concern during surgery was the performance of my anesthetist, because those doctors available to give anesthetics for me had not had a lot of experience or training in anesthesia. I had, as an intern, satisfactorily given a number of open drop ether and spinal anesthetics, and had given intravenous sodium pentothal for minor procedures. At first I believed that most interns had done the same during their internships, but soon learned that this was not so. When he came to town to practice Dr. Herman VanArk had had no "hands-on" experience in giving anesthetics The first time that he ever gave a general anesthetic was during our first December in Eaton Rapids, when he gave open drop ether to a patient of mine for a routine appendectomy. He had trouble keeping that patient deeply anesthetized, and didn't tell me until it was over that, although he had studied the subject in medical school, that was the first time he had ever actually administered an anesthetic.

Dr. Bert VanArk had given anesthetics in the past, but did not seem to like doing it, so we seldom called upon him for anesthesia. Dr. Bert often called upon Dr. Ralph Wadley, an excellent surgeon from Lansing, to come to Eaton Rapids to operate on one of his patients. Dr. Bert usually acted as the assistant surgeon, while Dr. Herman or I gave the anesthetic. At that time we were only capable of administering (1) local anesthetic agents, which we used mostly for small minor surgeries and to repair small lacerations, (2) open drop ether administered through an ether mask, and (3) spinal anesthetics. We specifically avoided the use of chloroform, which had been popular before World War II, because it had been implicated in cases of severe liver damage.

Because I had given a number of anesthetics under supervision during my internship at Sparrow, and in the latter months of the internship I had been trusted to give some without supervision, my experience in anesthesia was well enough known that it gained me privileges in anesthesia in both hospitals in Lansing. In the military service when my unit was returning from overseas, I was the only doctor on shipboard who had had any experience in anesthesia, and there I administered open drop ether to a soldier for the successful removal of an acutely inflamed appendix which was about to rupture. With such a background it appeared that I was probably the best qualified in anesthesia of all of the doctors in town. It also appeared that I was perhaps the most qualified to do surgery.

When we started our partnership practice as the Stimson Medical Group, we discussed arrangements for anesthesia among ourselves. I assured my partners that I would be available to give anesthetics for them. They did little major surgery but instead invited various surgical specialists to operate in Eaton Rapids on their patients, while they assisted in the surgery. I encouraged Dr. Herman to study up on anesthesia and become the anesthetist for the group, and he soon developed an excellent expertise in open drop ether anesthesia (mostly for T & As) and spinal anesthesia. Later on, when Dr. Eber Sherman joined our group, he did both surgery and anesthesia, and his presence allowed our hospital practice to expand with increasingly less reliance on outside surgeons to do the major operations. Later, when Dr. O. S. Erhard joined the group, he also did both surgery and anesthesia.

T & A was a popular operation in the early years, and we did a lot of them under open ether anesthesia with an ether hook, which is a hook-shaped tube, which delivers ether vapor into the patient's open mouth during the procedure. Open drop ether using an ether mask was used for abdominal operations, and when properly given, was an excellent and safe anesthetic. The main drawback with it was that for abdominal surgery, a high degree of muscle relaxation was needed to allow for good exposure of the operative field. Muscle relaxation was especially important when it came time to close the abdomen, and was often critical to easily getting all of the abdominal contents back inside. With ether, the depth of the anesthesia determines the amount of muscle relaxation present, and the ideal amount of relaxation for an abdominal operation is attained at about the depth of anesthesia at which the patient stops breathing. We used the size of the patient's pupils in the eye to gauge the depth of anesthesia, and fortunately, with ether, these eye signs were very reliable. The patient's pupils dilate just before spontaneous breathing ceases. This was the signal to stop administering ether in order to let the patient breathe room air and thus lighten the level of anesthesia. Occasionally, if a patient actually stopped breathing, we would perform one or two chest compressions to evacuate some of the air in the lungs, which still contained ether vapor. Within half a minute, sufficient ether in the patient's system would be metabolized, the level of anesthesia would lighten, and the patient would start breathing again.

Spinal anesthesia, on the other hand, completely blocks pain sensation and paralyzes all muscles below whatever level of anesthesia has been produced. It requires a "spinal tap," which is the insertion of a long needle between two vertebrae in the lower back into the spinal canal and into the space, which holds the spinal fluid. Then, depending upon the level of anesthesia desired and the length of time needed, a pre-calculated amount of a local anesthetic or a combination of such anesthetics is injected at a rate designed to have it ultimately reach the desired height in the spinal canal. If the height of anesthesia reached the chest, the abdominal muscles became paralyzed, and conditions for abdominal operations became ideal. The diaphragm, the sheet-like muscle at the bottom of the chest with the critical functions of producing inspiration and controlling expiration, would not become paralyzed, however, because it is controlled by the phrenic nerve, which has its control center high up at the base of the brain. The most common problem with high spinal anesthesia was hypotension (low blood pressure). We always watched for it and used vasopressor drugs judiciously to keep the patient's blood pressure from going too low.

In our medical group we used a lot of spinal anesthesia, because it was well suited for much of the surgery that we did, which consisted mostly of gynecological surgery, inguinal hernia repair, and appendectomy. We even had the expertise and courage to use it for gallbladder operations from time to time, and there would occasionally be a short period of anxiety when patients reported loss of feeling up into the neck

In caesarian sections we chose to use spinal anesthesia exclusively, because general inhalation anesthesia presented a special problem for the baby about to be born. Also the surgery could be more easily done with spinal anesthesia. If we were to use ether, it would take a relatively long time to get the mother anesthetized deeply enough to open the abdomen painlessly, and by that time the baby would also be anesthetized to nearly the same degree, as was the mother. This often interfered with the spontaneous start of respiration on the part of the baby, and would require that intense resuscitative efforts be applied to revive the newborn baby. Spinal anesthesia also had its dangers in caesarian sections, but we could cope with them more easily. During spinal anesthesia the danger to the baby arises from the sudden paralysis of half or more of the mother's body. This normally and promptly produces a sharp drop in the mother's blood pressure, because the muscle fibers in the walls of the blood vessels, which control their expansion and contraction, also become paralyzed. All of those vessels dilate maximally at the same time and allow the mothers blood to stagnate in them. The physiological effect is about the same as if about half of the mother's circulating blood volume were suddenly removed. This always causes her blood pressure to drop suddenly and significantly, and is also bad for the baby in the uterus because it markedly reduces the blood flowing to it from the mother, and decreases the amount of oxygen available for the baby's use through the placental circulation. To avoid this situation we developed a routine that worked very well. The surgeon who was to do the caesarian section always administered the spinal tap and injected the anesthetic agent. That way he would be already surgically scrubbed, and needed only to change gloves and gown and join his already prepared surgical team which in the meantime prepared the mother's abdomen and applied the sterile surgical drapes. He could then proceed immediately with the operation. As soon as the spinal anesthetic was injected, the anesthetist would give the mother a small dose of a vasopressor drug intramuscularly, large enough to keep the patient's blood pressure from falling too low, but small enough to keep it from going sky high as soon as the baby was born. All of this usually took a very few minutes, and usually the baby was extracted from the uterus within five or six minutes of the administration of the spinal anesthetic. Then, after the baby was out, if the mother wanted to be put to sleep for the rest of the operation, the anesthetist obliged. In actual practice very few mothers requested to be put to sleep.

The first modern innovation in anesthesia came to Eaton Rapids sometime just before 1950, and changed our obstetrical practice markedly. Until then anesthesia for childbirth consisted of whiffs of ether given by the nurse, after the patient had had a small dose of the synthetic narcotic, Demerol. Episiotomy, which is an incision through the perineum to enlarge the birth outlet, was repaired under local anesthesia. An anesthetic solution, usually Novocaine, was injected directly in and about the wound, and produced a very satisfactory anesthesia. I learned the procedure for "saddle block" spinal anesthesia in New York, and was first to use it in Eaton Rapids. The anesthetic agent used was Nupercaine, which was chosen for its long lasting action. To make the nupercaine solution substantially heavier than spinal fluid it was dissolved in a dextrose (sugar) solution. With the mother sitting upright, the calculated dose of anesthetic agent in its sugar solution was slowly injected into the spinal canal, and she was kept upright for a full minute afterward to allow the injected anesthetic solution to sink to the bottom of the spinal canal where the anesthetic effect was desired. Then for the next fifteen minutes or so the mother was placed on her back with a slight upward tilt to her trunk and her head up on a pillow. This was done in order to keep the anesthetic agent down in the lower end of the spinal canal until all of it became fixed in the nerve tissues.

Saddle block anesthesia was great for our obstetrical practices. It relieved most, but not quite all, of the pain involved in the labor contractions, but did not stop the uterine contractions, as a higher spinal or a general inhalation anesthetic would do. It was usually administered when labor was well established with a substantially dilated cervix, coinciding with the time when the really severe labor pains usually begin. Then with the mother more relaxed, the cervix would often dilate more rapidly, because the dilation process was not hindered by the patient straining or bearing down and cramming the whole uterus down into the pelvis. Usually the anesthetic effect lasted long enough for delivery to take place, and there would still be enough left for the repair of an episiotomy afterward.

Some years after we began using saddle block anesthesia, continuous caudal anesthesia became popular for both surgery and obstetrics. During labor continuous caudal provided an even greater relief of pain than did saddle block. It differed from a spinal anesthetic in that the needle was inserted into the spine, not into the spinal canal, which contains the spinal fluid, but between the tissue layers covering the brain and spinal cord, and the needle was left in place there. Only very tiny doses of anesthetic were needed, but they had to be repeated at intervals depending upon the recurrence of pain. This meant that a physician or a trained anesthetist had to practically remain at the bedside. Because the administration of the saddle block spinal anesthetic was included in our normal fee for our obstetrical cases, we felt that most of our patients would turn down the significant extra expense for an anesthetist at the bedside even if we could get one, and we neither encouraged nor did continuous caudals in our practice.

Significant changes in anesthesia also occurred in our operating rooms. Its evolution received a boost one day when Dr. Sherman was doing a caesarian section and I was serving as the anesthetist. He made the usual low transverse incision in the uterus, and delivered the baby without difficulty. He then expressed the placenta and confirmed that it was intact and whole. Then when he clamped the upper and lower edges of the uterine incision preparing to close it, a strong gush of blood came from the left side of the pelvis. There was so much blood that he could not see or find exactly where it was coming from. There was concern that the main uterine artery had been damaged. He tried hard to find the source of the bleeding, and quickly asked for help, so I told him to put a large laparotomy pack into the left side of the pelvis and hold it there while I scrubbed in to see what I could do. When, gowned and gloved, I finally got into the operative field it was obvious that the pack had done a good job of temporarily stemming the blood flow. After removing the pack I was able to quickly deliver the entire uterus out of the abdomen, and with my hand now behind it, I was able to stop the hemorrhage with pressure between my thumb and fingers. This allowed me to inspect the uterine attachments, and I was relieved to see that the main uterine artery was not damaged, but several of the large branches coming off of it had been cut or torn during the delivery of the baby. After the careful placement of three chromic catgut suture ligatures, the excessive bleeding was well controlled, and I could now clearly see and identify the uterine incision, its interior surface and its exterior surface. The crisis was over! I was able to do a normal closure of the uterus and then of the abdomen, while Dr Sherman monitored the state of the patient's anesthesia. When we estimated blood loss at the end of the operation it appeared that she had lost only a little more than the amount she would have lost in a normal vaginal delivery. Her condition remained good, and her eventual recovery was uneventful.

This experience so unnerved Dr. Sherman that he immediately announced, "This is it! I'm not doing any more surgery. I'll stick to anesthesia!"

Dr. Sherman kept his word. He studied anesthesia in detail. He studied heart disease and electrocardiography in detail. Before long he was reading the electrocardiograms for all of us in the group. I don't know if he ever became board certified in anesthesiology, but it is my opinion the he was certainly qualified to be board certified. Later in his career he attended anesthesia seminars and meetings, and even occasionally taught a class at the Michigan State University Medical School. He was the first of our group to be able to intubate a patient, and eventually intubated many patients, including small children and babies, seemingly with ease. It was through his efforts that the anesthesia services at the Eaton Rapids Community Hospital not only stayed up to date, but flourished. As he learned new things and started new practices, he also taught them to me, and when I retired I was still able to give a good, modern anesthetic.

The next innovation in anesthesia came when the hospital under Dr. Sherman's guidance obtained a modern anesthesia machine. Now we were able to give GOE (gas, oxygen, ether) anesthesia. The administration of the anesthetic agents was more precise and was completely controllable with the machine. We could now avoid the choking and gagging caused by ether by putting the patient to sleep with nitrous oxide (laughing gas) or a small intravenous dose of a short acting barbiturate. Then ether was added with the patient already asleep, to take over the main burden of the anesthesia. There was an ether evaporator on the machine through which passed the gases to be breathed, and I was constantly surprised by the small amount of ether needed to put a patient into deep anesthesia and keep him accurately at that level.

Next there came two innovations that put the practice of administering anesthetics far ahead of previous practices. They were the standard use of endotracheal intubation, and the use of paralyzing agents such as succinylcholine and the South American arrow poison, curare. In practice the patient was given a preoperative sedative, and after it had taken effect, he was taken to the operating room, where an intravenous line was placed in an arm vein and kept open with a slow drip of an intravenous solution. Next he would receive enough sodium pentothal (short-acting barbiturate) intravenously to lightly anesthetize him and render him unconscious. Then he would receive, all at once, an intravenous dose of the paralytic agent. I liked succinylcholine, which has no antidote, but which is rapidly broken down by an enzyme normally present in the body called cholinesterase.

At this point in the proceedings we have a patient sound asleep and completely paralyzed, therefore not breathing. We now rapidly place an endotracheal tube into his trachea, seal it in with the balloon that is there for that purpose, and connect the endotracheal tube to the anesthesia machine. Now we can breathe for the patient manually by squeezing the rubber bag on the machine to push air or a gas and oxygen mixture into his lungs. The gas mixture might be 75% nitrous oxide and 25% oxygen (air is about 20 % oxygen), but it could contain almost any kind of gaseous anesthetic agent. When, in about six or seven minutes the effect of the slug of succinylcholine wears off and the patient begins breathing by himself, we drip a dilute solution of succinylcholine into the open intravenous line, and adjust it rate of flow so that the patient's muscles are partially paralyzed but he remains breathing on his own.

The patient is now ready for surgery and the anesthetist finds himself in a much calmer situation. He does not need to worry about putting the patient into the deep stages of anesthesia, and thus avoids the dangers of anesthetic overdosage. His only concern with depth of anesthesia is to be sure that the patient remains unconscious. He can avoid any threat of anesthetic "poisoning" by using small doses of several agents, and as long as the patient remains unconscious, he can accommodate the surgeon with whatever degree of muscle relaxation is needed by increasing and decreasing the flow of the succinylcholine drip, even to the point of complete paralysis, during which time he breathes for the patient by repeatedly squeezing the bag on the anesthetic machine. After the abdomen is closed the succinylcholine drip is stopped and the patient soon breathes by himself again. During the surgery he never was under deep, deep anesthesia, so he is quick to wake up. Some of my cases have been so wide-awake by the time they were wheeled out of the operating room, that I believe they could have walked.

In the ensuing years other innovations for anesthesia came into the picture. They did not affect the general principles of anesthesiology, but were designed to better and more accurately control the anesthesia administration and monitor the patient's condition. In the beginning of the era of muscle relaxants we monitored blood pressure with a cuff on the patients' arm and a stethoscope taped onto the skin below it. The anesthetist took blood pressures intermittently and recorded them on the anesthetic record. Likewise he periodically took the patient's pulse rate and recorded it. This was usually done by counting the carotid pulse in the neck, but some of us slipped a catheter through the patient's nose into his esophagus, and by attaching the catheter to a stethoscope, we could hear the patient's heartbeat continuously. Subsequent developments include cardiac monitoring during surgery, which shows the anesthetist an EKG (electrocardiograph) tracing on a screen. Modern monitors also show the blood pressure, respiratory rate, and the degree of oxygenation of the blood. Many other things can be and are monitored during anesthesia.

Because I have been away from it for eighteen years now, when I see the array of monitors and gadgets in the operating rooms of today I am a bit overwhelmed. Anesthesia has evolved a long way from the day I started out with a preoperative sedative, an ether mask, and a can of ether with a safety pin stuck through its seal. Yet I still take some pride in the belief that I could still administer a safe and satisfactory anesthetic today, using only those things that were then available.

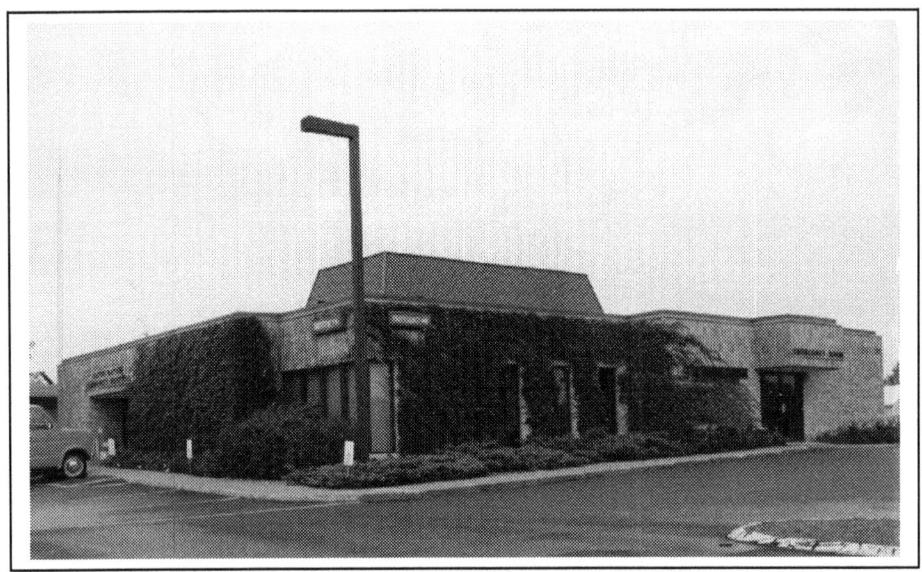

This is how the Eaton Rapids Community Hospital looked after the Emergency Room was brought upstairs out of the basement and enlarged, the kitchen was rebuilt in the basement, and a new lobby and gift shop were added. At the far right the main entrance of the hospital has become the new entrance to the emergency suite. The new main entrance is seen at the far left. The picture was taken from the parking area at the corner of Main Street and Spicerville Highway.

CHAPTER XVIII

EMERGENCY SERVICES

When I arrived to begin my medical practice there was no formal emergency service in Eaton Rapids. The Lansing and Jackson Hospitals operated emergency rooms, but they were miles away. Closest was the Emergency Room at St. Lawrence Hospital, a distance of some 15 miles, and that was a bit far for the injured patient to go to have only a few stitches placed or to have a simple fracture treated. In severe cases, however, when it was obvious that more extensive medical care would be needed than was available in our small town, it was common practice for one of the local ambulances to take the patient directly to one of the larger city emergency rooms. Even then it was not certain that there would be a doctor on duty, because it was the common practice of the day for individual doctors on the hospital staff to be on call for emergency room coverage, and to be there only when called to take care of whatever emergency may have come in. During my internship at Sparrow Hospital in Lansing, there was always an intern present in the building, who could usually be in the emergency room in a minute if needed. Most of the time the intern, who was a licensed physician, treated the emergency, and referred the patient to his own personal doctor's office for follow-up. I know this for certain, because I was one of those interns. Sometimes a telephone message that the arrival of a serious case was on its way would be received ahead of time, and the intern on duty could then alert the proper specialist as to when and what type of case was expected. Those emergency patients that required hospital admission were admitted into the care of one of the regular staff doctors, who took full charge of the case. However the intern who was on duty when the patient arrived also followed the patient's course of treatment and progress in the hospital.

For most emergencies in the Eaton Rapids area it was common practice to call the family doctor by phone, and if he could not be reached, to call another doctor or take the patient to Stimson Hospital, where the nurse on duty would summon a doctor to see him. Actually the first rudimentary emergency room in Eaton Rapids came into being when the Stimson Medical Group moved their offices into the hospital, and used the large examining room, which had been walled off from the lobby, to care for emergency cases. When the room was not being used for an emergency, it was my office examining room. As it began being used more and more for emergencies, we started to keep more and more emergency supplies there, and added more emergency equipment from time to time. Each day one doctor from our Stimson Medical Group kept himself available to treat emergencies on call, and all of us rotated through this duty. Single medical records as used in the Group clinic were also used for emergencies, and most of the emergency patients returned to us for follow-up care. Only occasionally was it necessary to write a letter to an out-of-town doctor describing what we had done for his patient. This was the first, rudimentary emergency room set-up in Eaton Rapids.

Occasionally there were injuries, which occurred to high school athletes. Stitches were occasionally needed during football season, and I remember occasionally stitching up lacerations sustained by members of both home and visiting teams during games. There were night games, and some athletic injuries occurred at night. There were strains, sprains and suspected fractures, which were often diagnosed handily because the x-ray machine was right there close to our "emergency room." We could readily answer many of the questions of diagnosis that we faced.

Eaton Rapids got its first real Emergency Room in the summer of 1957 when Stimson Hospital closed in favor of the new Eaton Rapids Community Hospital. The emergency room was located in the surgical wing at the back of the hospital. A long concrete ramp rose up from the parking lot pavement to the level of the main floor of the hospital and joined a concrete slab porch. Double doors opened from the porch into a wide hall, and fifteen feet beyond was the doorway of the emergency room. There was also room on the porch for ambulances to unload their patient carts directly on to the porch. Alongside this ramp, between it and the main wall of the hospital, was another ramp that was steeper, which led down to a basement entrance under the porch.

The emergency room itself was set up like a minor surgery, and was actually so well equipped that it was often actually used as a minor surgery room for short operative procedures. Along one wall were cabinets to hold medicines and supplies, and there was a writing desk fastened to the wall where the emergency room records were written. The autoclave for sterilizing instruments and surgical packs was only a few feet away across the hall in one direction, and x-ray was only about 40 feet down the hall past the main hospital nursing station. Everything was handy.

When this new emergency room opened for patient care, we began using separate emergency medical records, a separate one for each emergency room visit. The originals were kept in the hospital records department, and a duplicate was sent to the patient's doctor's office. There was also a nurse on duty in the emergency room, but when the room was not busy she could help out on the main hospital floor. The main nursing station was located only about 20 feet from the emergency room door, which made shifting back and forth easy. This arrangement worked very well, with the surgery nursing staff running it in the daytime, an additional nurse running it for the afternoon shift, and the night staff of the hospital covering it from 11:00 p.m. until 7:00 a.m.

Even before the new hospital opened, Stimson Medical Group made a decision to build new offices nearby. The group bought several acres of apple orchard across Spicerville Highway from the hospital, and construction began shortly after the hospital opened. When they moved into their new offices the STIMSON MEDICAL GROUP changed its name to EATON RAPIDS MEDICAL CLINIC. After the move it was even easier to cover the emergency room, and the move also prompted an increase in use of the emergency room for minor surgical procedures. Except for occasionally being crowded this emergency care system continued to work well.

A few years later when the new Obstetrical Wing was added to the hospital building it gave us an opportunity to upgrade and enlarge the emergency room and the services offered. In order to do this a new emergency room was built in the newly constructed basement of the new addition at the southernmost end of the building. This basement was not set very deep in the ground, and a long concrete ramp with a very shallow grade, about eight feet wide and covered by a fiberglass canopy, led onto the basement floor from the street level outside. We also had to build another outside entrance at the other end of the addition where the new joined the old, and in this area we also installed an elevator large enough to easily move beds and patients between floors. With the emergency room gone from the surgical wing changes in the surgical area were also made. The old emergency room was divided into doctors' and nurses' dressing rooms, and the old doctor's dressing room was remodeled into a second operating room.

In the new emergency room there were two large cubicles, each completely fitted out so that two patients could be accommodated simultaneously, and there was in addition a complete private examining room. There was also another large room, which was set up for physiotherapy services, in which we also applied plasters and casts. There were chairs along the hallway, which was then used as a waiting area.

After this second emergency room was put into operation, we had little trouble with inspectors and regulators, and the service itself worked smoothly. I was deeply involved because from the beginning I had "fallen" into the position of Chief of Emergency Services, and was kept informed of all problems that arose. I remember only one time that I "squared off" with a pharmacy inspector who was sent to inspect the drugs we kept in the emergency room. We were fully aware that the law required accurate records to be kept of all narcotic drugs used, and that those substances had to be kept under lock and key. Ours were, as well as some other drugs we considered dangerous or expensive. The inspector looked into our unlocked cabinets and soon pulled out a multiple dose vial of a non-narcotic drug, claiming that it should have been locked up because it was a restricted drug. As proof he pointed to a small circle surrounding a capital "R." on the label. Here was another example of an incompetent inspector. He didn't believe me when I told him that the symbol stood for "Registered Trade Mark", and was there because the drug company was protecting its trade name for the medicine. I don't know whether or not he reported us for this "infraction," but we didn't receive any citations from the drug people that year. My memories of this second emergency room are good ones. It seemed to operate very well.

The third emergency room to be created in the hospital is the one still in operation at the time of this writing. Its development was really triggered by the hospital's need for a larger, more conveniently located laboratory area. When the remodeling was complete, the laboratory had moved into what had been the kitchen, the hospital lobby had been enlarged and was now a new emergency suite, with four cubicles on one side of the hall and a private examining room on the other. The main hospital entrance was placed off to the South and entered a vestibule with stairs to the basement where the new kitchen was built. The vestibule also opened into a new lobby area with attached gift shop. The rest of the old and a part of the new construction became a registration area.

It is my recollection that this third emergency room also worked very well, and that there were a number of times during which I was involved with emergency patients that I was especially thankful to have the extra space.

CHAPTER XIX

THE CORONER SYSTEM

In early times the funeral directors in Eaton County acted as coroner and signed the official Death Certificate whenever a newly deceased person had had no medical treatment and there was no doctor to sign it. The funeral directors also determined the cause of death, and a review of those old death certificates turns up some amazing diagnoses. Elderly people often died of indigestion, but we now know that most of them had coronary artery disease and died of coronary occlusion and myocardial infarction (heart attacks). Whenever a cause of death was not obviously apparent, the funeral director often chose "heart failure" or "natural causes." It seemed to me as if it would have been easy to murder someone in those old times, and get away with it. The true cause of death would have been easy to hide, and the victim might have officially died of a "heart attack" or "natural causes."

The legislature of the State of Michigan abruptly ended this practice with laws that required each county to have, as its coroner, a Medical Examiner who was a physician. Eaton County was obliged to hire one. The laws included provisions for investigating deaths, and required the performance of autopsies (post-mortem examinations in which the inside of the body is also examined) in all cases where the cause of death was suspected to be foul play, or in which there was a reasonable possibility that, because of the death, a lawsuit would result. County governments did not like this at all, because autopsies had to be done by medical specialists who were pathologists or forensic pathologists, and the cost seemed expensive in the eyes of most county commissioners.

During the early years under the new system the story began circulating that an indigent hitchhiker had unexpectedly dropped dead at the roadside just a few feet inside the county line. The first sheriff department officers to arrive at he scene were from the county in which the body was lying, and they immediately dragged the body a few feet across the county line. This changed the county in which the death had officially occurred, so that the neighboring county would be required to pay for the autopsy that followed.

Medical examiners also had to be knowledgeable of such things as the preservation of evidence and other legal issues involved. Educational seminars periodically became available for them to attend.

Fortunately, most of the deaths in Eaton County occurred to people who were under the care of a physician, and there were generally no problems in determining the cause of death. The law stated that if the deceased had been seen (attended) by the attending physician within the 24-hour period immediately prior to death, the physician must complete and sign the death certificate. If the time period was longer than 24 hours, the county medical examiner was responsible for determining the cause of death, and completing and signing the death certificate. However, in most cases, if the deceased had been under the care of a physician or was a regular patient of a physician, the medical examiner would call that physician, discuss the deceased's health problems, and the two doctors together would determine the cause of death. The medical examiner would then complete and sign the death certificate.

Problems arose in cases in which there had been no attending physician. Those cases required investigation, and the County Medical Examiner had to arrive upon the scene, carry out the investigation, and give his permission before the body could be moved. If any suspicion of foul play arose, the sheriff had to be notified, a report had to be written, an autopsy had to be ordered, and police officers summoned to the scene if they were not already there. Deaths occurring in automobile accidents often had suspicious nuances, and in many of them, ensuing lawsuits were likely to follow.

Under the Medical Examiner System I was quite satisfied that no longer could one easily "get away with murder." There seemed to be a problem however in that the doctor who was the medical examiner was kept hopping. He soon felt that he was overworked, and wanted to quit the position. Even with a physician assistant there seemed to be too much to do. So at a meeting of the Eaton County Medical Society almost all of the doctors living and practicing within the county agreed to become Deputy Medical Examiners, and act for the County Medical Examiner in the areas in which they practiced. We all received educational material explaining the job, and were duly sworn in. I learned that the medical examiner was a powerful political figure, and was legally the only person in the county that could put the sheriff under arrest.

Under this arrangement one of the deputies went to the death scenes of what was labeled a "coroner's case," and did the investigating, reporting, and signed the certificates. None of us liked this work. It often entailed getting out of bed in the middle of the night, driving to the scene of an accident, or to the bedroom of some old person who had died in his sleep, and then, the next day, completing a number of reports and signing the death certificate. For this we were paid $30 per case, regardless of how many hours of investigation had been necessary.

While acting as deputy medical examiner I was exposed to some unusual cases. My regular patients and people who were my friends did not become coroner's cases. They had medical histories with me or with their family doctor, and when this information was considered, it was not difficult to decide upon a cause of death. The medical examiner cases that I handled were all deaths of strangers to me, and after the passage of so many years, I do not remember a single name.

The coroner's case that I think about most often is the one that troubled me the most at the time that it happened. It was a sheer foolish waste of the life of a young man and woman. Their deaths occurred in the village of Dimondale, which is located about ten miles North of Eaton Rapids.

This young man had worked in one of the General Motors automobile plants in Lansing, and sometime previously had claimed that he had injured his back at work. After going through the gamut of examinations, treatments, and efforts at rehabilitation, he sued the company. After lengthy legal proceedings, during which time he didn't work, he was finally offered a lump sum settlement, which he accepted. The first thing he did with the money was to buy the biggest, most powerful Harley-Davidson motorcycle available. He had taken possession of the machine that very day, and to celebrate the occasion he spent the entire evening with his girl friend in a tavern in Dimondale. When the tavern closed at 2:00 a.m., they left, both riding on the Harley, and followed the route of some other motorcycles belonging to friends who had left the tavern ahead of them.

About half a mile from the tavern the road curved sharply to the left, and the outside edge of the curve was guarded by a low metal guardrail. The motorcycle on which the two were riding at a high rate of speed apparently struck a guardrail post almost squarely, which stopped the machine almost instantly. The two riders were projected upward over the guardrail, and while flying through the air in a horizontal position the man's body struck a stout, steel sign post, one of a pair that held up a large road sign. The post hit the body at about the lower edge of the rib cage, and almost cut it in half. The girl's body flew up over the sign and into a stand of stout saplings about 50 yards beyond it. Her injuries were not so immediately apparent, but when I arrived at the scene she, too, was dead. The causes of death were obvious, so I authorized removal of the bodies to the local funeral parlor and followed after them. There I took blood samples from both bodies, and turned them over to the police before I left to go home. The following afternoon I finished filling in and signed the death certificates.

Another coroner's case that I attended was a death in an auto accident which happened four or five miles North of Eaton Rapids in a construction zone in the winter time while State Highway M-99 was being rebuilt into a four lane highway. There was snow on the ground and the road was slippery. Excessive speed appears to have been the cause of the accident. Only one older model car was involved, which had apparently left the road at the bottom of a hill, bounced off of several construction-site objects and ended up upright in the median at right angles to the road. The deceased was an elderly woman, who was markedly overweight. She was still sitting upright in the right front seat of the car, --- held there by the still buckled seat belt. The car door next to which she had been sitting had been pushed in, but it still opened, and I could get to her without difficulty. I arrived at the scene about thirty minutes after the accident had happened, and when I examined the body it was already getting cold, despite the fact that she was wearing heavy winter clothing. This led me to believe that she had died very quickly, but I was unable to tell specifically what had killed her. Out there in the car I could see no external signs of injury from which she could have died, and later in the funeral home there was still not much to indicate how much she had been injured internally. I wanted an autopsy, but the sheriff said that the incident was purely an accident with no evidence of foul play, and the county commission refused my request. So I guessed, and signed her out as having died of massive internal hemorrhage due to trauma, because I visualized that her aorta had possibly been split open lengthwise by the heavy blow to the car, which had dented in the door next to which she was sitting.

In another coroner's case the deceased was one of my regular patients, and the physician coroner called to consult with me regarding the possible causes of death. The story went that the deceased had run his pickup truck through a stop sign on a rural road into a county highway, and had been struck broadside by another vehicle. He had died before he could be removed from the truck, and there was some question about whether or not the other driver could have avoided the collision or not. My patient was considered old, but apparently healthy, and not under treatment for advanced disease of any kind. Certainly he was old enough to have "hardening of the arteries," but I was not treating him for heart disease, and he had never had a stroke. There were rumblings that somebody was ready to sue, so we decided to insist upon an autopsy before signing the death certificate. I was able to attend the autopsy, which revealed that over half of the dead man's heart muscle was probably dead before the accident. This was later confirmed by microscopic examination. The cause of death was a massive myocardial infarction. The man was dead at the wheel of his truck before it even reached the stop sign.

Another sad accident to which I was summoned as a deputy medical examiner occurred on a farm some eight or nine miles Southwest of town. The accident had occurred on the farm woodlot where the middle-aged farmer was clearing out tree stumps with a large farm tractor. Technicians from the EMS (Emergency Medical Service) were there when I arrived, and had already determined that the man was dead. It was early spring with some snow still on the ground, so I could not drive out into the woodlot. Therefore I accompanied the EMT's (Emergency Medical Technicians) back to the scene of the accident on foot. We soon arrived, and it was easy to tell what had happened. The deceased was still on the rough ground, with a part of his body still compressed under the tractor. The tractor had no cab on it, and was lying upside-down with its wheels directed toward the sky. A long steel cable had been wrapped around a large stump, and then hitched to the tractor, but the connection had been made much too high on the back end of the tractor! It was above the level of the rear axle, so that when the farmer had tried to pull the stump out of the ground, the tractor went forward, but was held back by the cable. However, the wheels continued forward, forcing the tractor's axle out from under the cable attachment. The result was that the nose of the tractor rose rapidly up into the air, the tractor flipped over on to its top, crushing the driver and killing him quickly. I was satisfied as to the cause of death, and gave permission to move the body, but didn't stay to see it done. I believe that the funeral director's crew and some neighboring farmers eventually righted the tractor and extracted the body. This farmer and his family had been patients of Dr. Herman VanArk, and I knew them casually. It was hard for me to go into that house and explain to the man's wife what had happened, but I am glad that I was able to do it. I hope it helped to make the loss more bearable.

There were other coroner's cases also. I'm glad that there weren't many. I remember only a few. There was the suicide from carbon monoxide poisoning which occurred in a farmyard. The despondent young man had hooked a large hose to the exhaust pipe of the car and had run it inside. He did have the cherry red lips and pink cheeks we read about in medical school. There was the shotgun blast into the mouth of an old man, which caused instant death. Most coroner's stories are not pleasant.

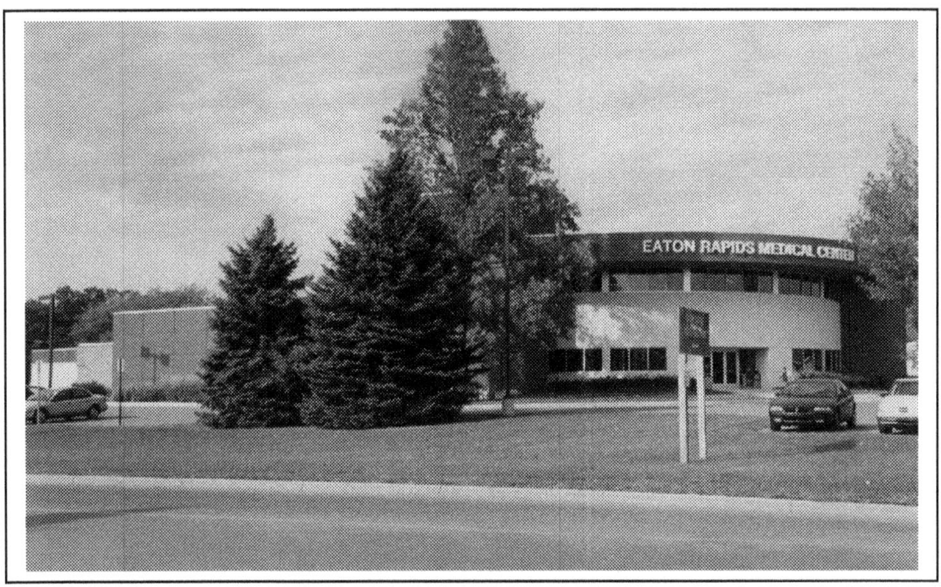

***EATON RAPIDS MEDICAL CENTER** as it appears today in the year 2002. The main entrance is new and the large area on the floor above is being remodeled into a **WELLNESS CENTER**. The emergency entrance is still in the same place, but is now shielded from Main Street by a brick wall and an overhead canopy. At the far left the car is parked in the parking lot for the emergency room. Beyond that is another parking lot for patients and visitors. Beyond that, across Spicerville Highway is the former Eaton Rapids Medical Clinic building, which is now part of the Medical Center.*

CHAPTER XX

HOUSECALL ADVENTURES

From the very beginning of my practice I received requests for house calls, and in my first twenty or so years I made many of them. It did not take me long to realize that house calls used up a lot of time without providing an equivalent in benefit to my patients. Most of the house calls that I made were truly not necessary and were not very productive. They were also not fun for me, but I continued to make them cheerfully because it was the thing for a small town doctor to do, and it was expected by my patients.

The main reasons for my less than enthusiastic feelings about house calls involved time and money. Depending upon how far I had to drive, a house call required three to five times as much time as it took to care for a patient in the office, but I could not bring myself to charge three to five times the cost of an office call. The office call was $3.00; but the house call was only $5.00,--- sometimes $6.00 or even $7.00, if the drive to get there was long. Then there was the ever-present knowledge that I could do more for the patient in the office or the hospital. Many times have I gone out to a home, to find that it was necessary for me to tell the patient to come in to the office or hospital for some specific procedure, such as an x-ray, or a special treatment for his complaint. This usually left me with the feeling that I had done nothing for the patient, and sometimes led me to absorb the cost of the house call into the charge for whatever was done later in the office or hospital. As time went on these time and cost benefit differences became ever greater, and eventually honest house calls became financially impossible for both doctor and many patients.

Before my office practice had grown to capacity, I sometimes made house calls during the day, but my days soon became so filled with hospital and office hours that I could only make house calls in the evenings. Rarely could I squeeze one in here and there during the day. Evening house calls became routine, and were a part of my life for many years. I never knew the luxury of an eight-hour workday.

My stories involving house calls do not appear here in chronological order, because for most of them my memory of the date and time of occurrence is completely gone. I don't remember people's names very well and remember their stories mainly because something medically unusual occurred, or because there was something humorous connected with them.

A Dermatology Lesson

One afternoon, I think it was in December of my first year in practice, I had not been very busy in the office and was finished early. I was therefore able to make a house call before dinner to an area into which I had not previously gone. The directions took me East of town a far distance across Highway US-127, and before I reached the place I knew that this was too far for me to come, and that this would be the last time I would drive this far on a house call.

The patient was a middle-aged farmer. He complained of a sore throat, and after I had prescribed for it and was ready to leave, his wife asked if I would please see Grandpa, who was out behind the barn suffering from an itchy skin problem.

So I went with her, and there, behind the barn, sticking up out of a huge pile of what appeared to be rotting manure, was a man's head, wearing a large woolen winter cap with earflaps open and flying. This was Grandpa. He told me that he had dug a hole in the manure pile, stripped naked, crawled in, and covered himself with it. This had eased his itching almost immediately and now it was all but gone. He said he was comfortable, and added,

"It's nice and warm in here too!"

This development surprised me, and I had to stop and think about it. What was expected of me?

Dermatology (Diseases of the Skin) had not been my best subject in medical school. Skin rashes, especially those shown in textbooks or on a screen with lectures, all seemed to look pretty much alike to me. I found it difficult to appreciate all of the nuances of the characteristics of the rash being described. I did however remember one pearl of dermatological wisdom about the treatment of chronic skin eruptions. ***"If it's a dry rash, wet it; if it's a wet rash dry it; if you don't know what it is soak it until it gets well!"***

I had the patient push aside some of the manure on his chest and shoulder, and I could see that he did indeed have a rash and there was evidence that he had scratched it. I didn't know what it was or what name to put to it. I asked if the skin had blistered or wept fluid, and he said that it had not. I thought that it was perhaps some kind of dry eczema, and noted that the patient was keeping it wet, albeit with rotting manure. He seemed to actually be doing the right thing. So I told him to stay where he was as long as he thought necessary, or until the rash cleared up. Then, after he had washed up, if he still itched he should try a healing, moisturizing lotion, and if necessary, oatmeal baths. Such baths were popular for itching at the time, and are still being used occasionally today.

I had collected my fee for the house call from my patient inside the house. I did not charge Grandpa anything at all.

Goose Attack

This house call occurred just before midnight on a winter night at a farm about three miles out of town. It was a clear night with a bright moon, and although it had not snowed for two or three days, there was still plenty of clean, white snow on the ground. The light of the nearly full moon reflecting from it lit up the landscape so that it was almost as bright as day.

Making a house call to a farm usually involved driving into a farmyard and parking as close as practical to the back door of the farmhouse. This time I had to park about 40 feet from the door of a woodshed, which was attached to the back of the house.

Almost every farm had at least one dog, and for the most part these dogs had the run of their farmyards. I never had problems with them. Whenever I would step out of my car and a strange dog was nearby, I would carry my medical bag in hand, and as the dog came up to me I would hold it out toward the dog. Usually the dog would stop and carefully smell the bag. Once satisfied the dog would wander off or trot alongside of me as I walked up to the house. This time there was the usual dog in the yard to greet me, but he did not linger long, because from behind the barn came a loud noise composed of hissing, honking and squawking. I had just time to turn and see a flock of huge geese came charging around the corner of the barn. I didn't think that my medical bag would deter them, and I had in the past been warned that geese could be vicious in their attacks, so I made haste toward the back door of the house.

As did many in the area, this farmhouse had a woodshed attached to the back of it. The door had been taken off at the hinges, and it was standing on its side across the open doorway inside the shed. I vaulted over it into the shed and was shocked to find that I did not land on solid ground. Whatever I had landed upon was soft and moved immediately. There began a loud squealing and grunting that I recognized as belonging to a pig. I was quickly airborne again, and bounded to the doorstep of the house. Fortunately the door was not locked, and I could enter the kitchen immediately. There was a light on in the room, and as I entered, I turned and looked back into the shed. There, indeed, was the biggest pig I had ever seen. I learned later that it was a sow weighing about six hundred pounds.

Now I found myself in what was obviously a kitchen. There was a peculiar odor in the room, and what appeared to be several hundred baby chicks were running all over the floor and peeping. A table leaf, which had been propped up on edge, stood across the doorway leading into a dining room, and kept them in the kitchen. I stepped over it and called out as I moved slowly through a dining room toward a living room or parlor. A woman's voice answered, and in seconds a middle-aged woman with a large envelope in her hand appeared in a doorway that led from the living room into a bedroom. Clad in somewhat soiled pajamas she ran up to me, opened the envelope, opened up its contents to a certain spot, and handed the whole thing to me, saying,

"Is this any good?"

It took only a few questions to learn the woman's name, and that she was not the patient's wife. From her appearance I mentally placed her into the populace category of "the unwashed." I looked at the papers she had handed to me, and recognized a life insurance policy on the life of the man who was about to become my patient. The insured value was $500. The woman had opened it to the page that showed the designation of the beneficiary, and there I read her name followed by the words, "a friend." After telling her that she would need to consult an insurance agent for the company to find that out, I asked about the patient. She showed me into the bedroom.

There in the bed was my patient, a man in his late sixties, having a lot of trouble breathing. Now the woman crawled back into the bed from which she had obviously arisen when I came in, and explained that she was getting cold.

Fortunately the diagnosis was easy to make. The patient was suffering with congestive heart failure, which I thought was probably due to arteriosclerotic heart disease. Although he denied being nauseated and was not vomiting, I gave him a diuretic medication by injection, watched him swallow a starter dose of digitalis, and left more digitalis with written instructions as to how to take it to effect a slow digitalization. A prescription for an oral diuretic completed the initial treatment program. Subsequently I saw him in the office a few times, and learned that the heart failure was difficult to control. He died soon afterward.

When I left the house the patient felt much better, and was breathing easily. I left via the front door, tiptoeing quietly back to my car, and keeping a wary eye out for geese.

Redecorating Anyone?

When I first moved to town James and Effie Fuller, a married couple about my age, lived on River Street. They had two young girls who were prone to having more than just colds in the winter. They often had laryngotracheobronchitis, which in non-medical jargon is old-fashioned croup. I did not make many housecalls to their home, but I do remember one in which both girls had the typical barking cough of croup. There were no medicines that cured it, but sooner or later the patients all got well. For relief of symptoms I recommended aspirin if needed for aching and fever, some cough medicine as needed to help control the often-painful cough, and the standard treatment, which was steam and vapor inhalation.

Various steamers, inhalers and croup tents were commonly being used, and physicians were often asked what to put into the water that was being used in them. Such things as Tincture of Benzoin, eucalyptus oil, menthol, and oil of peppermint were commonly recommended. Having been subjected to some of these treatments myself when I was small, I knew how sharp and acrid some of these smells could be, and I believed that they should be used in small concentrations, only enough to stimulate secretions in the respiratory system. I explained this to Effie, and told her that it was impossible to over-treat the children with water vapor, but if heat was being used to create the vapor, she must take care not to overheat the children into a state of hyperthermia. It didn't matter much what was put into the water as long as it smelled nice.

Effie, being a no nonsense person, decided that instead of erecting a croup tent for each child, she would turn their bedroom into one big one, using multiple steamers to assure that enough water vapor would be produced to provide good treatment. The next morning the Fullers were shocked to see that the wallpaper in the bedroom had been steamed off of the walls and was coming down in rolls. Since that day James and Effie have remained among my most liked friends, and as the years went by we would occasionally recall, with a chuckle, this night when the wallpaper came down.

Bogged Down

During the annual spring thaw the appearance of the landscape around Eaton Rapids would change quickly. As the snow rapidly melted away, the farmland became very wet, and we would see standing water in places everywhere. In the early days most of the county roads were not paved. Some were decently graveled with good drainage, but many were still quite primitive. In the spring many of these became quagmires of mud and gravel, and one often chose to avoid them.

This was the situation when at about two o'clock in the morning I was awakened by a phone call with a plea for help. An elderly man had not been able to urinate for over twelve hours and was in great pain. The story sounded like he had acute urinary retention. When the bladder becomes rapidly overfilled, it also becomes very painful. I agreed to come, dressed immediately and began the trip to the patient's home, but before leaving town I stopped at my office to pick up some sterile catheters and sterile rubber gloves.

It had been raining for hours and the snow was practically gone, but there was still frost in the ground, which gave the gravel roads some solidity and made them relatively easy to travel. In spite of that I took a slightly longer way to get to the patient's house in order to take advantage of better roads. When I arrived I drove into the farmyard and parked near the back door of the house.

As expected, I found the patient to have a markedly distended urinary bladder, and was able to bring quick relief by inserting a catheter, which I taped in place. I checked for other problems, and found a very much-enlarged prostate gland, but it did not seem to have any of the signs of cancer. I then stayed by the bedside to drain the bladder slowly, in increments, until it was empty. The urine was clear and looked quite normal, but I warned about the dangers of infection from an indwelling catheter, then told the patient and his wife that I would refer him to an urologist, whom he should visit in Lansing for necessary treatment. I would have someone from my office make an appointment for him, and call him to let him know when it was scheduled and where to go. Then I placed a clamp on the indwelling catheter, and showed him how to open it to let the urine drain out at intervals.

When I left the farmhouse it was still raining, and as I walked toward my car, it seemed to be small and quite low. Then I noticed that the frost in the ground must have thawed. All four wheels had sunk to the wheel hubs into the mud, and the car frame was resting in the mud. There was nothing to do but call for help. So back into the house I went.

It took about forty-five minutes for the tow truck to arrive from town, driven by a man I am sure I knew, but now I have forgotten who he was. I remember only that he was very cheerful, and had me pulled out of the farmyard and on to the road in a short time. Then I remember that he gave me a bill for his services. It was for $15. The irony of the situation struck me. I had just made a house call some seven miles into the country during which I gave away a brand new catheter and clamp, and charged the patient $7. The cost of that house call to me was: $15 for the tow truck, about $2.50 for the cost of driving my car, and about $2 for the catheter. And I also had lost half of a night's sleep.

A Birth in "Squalor City"

At about 4:00 a.m. one morning late in the spring, there came a vigorous knock on my front door. I awoke, arose from my bed, went downstairs and answered the door. There was a young man standing there who appeared to be desperate. He begged me to come to his house to see his wife who was having terrible pain "in the belly" and looked "awful sick." I agreed to go, and when I found out approximately where he lived, I said I would follow him there in my car. I followed his old wreck of a car some ten or twelve miles, and somewhere South of Springport we arrived at his house. Daylight was barely beginning to show as we parked about forty feet from the front door. He led the way to the door and in the path to it we had to climb up over a mound, which was about three feet high and ten feet from the door. As I climbed over it, I noticed that it was really a mound of garbage in which I recognized eggshells and grapefruit rinds. Apparently it was a household habit to just heave the garbage out through the front door.

When we reached the doorway, I saw that there was no door there, but an old blanket had been hung over it to try to keep out the cold. Inside, I immediately noticed the bare earth underfoot, and realized that the house was without a floor. It was essentially one big room with several posts holding up a dirty ceiling. Some boxes and furnishings standing around gave the illusion that it was divided into rooms. In one corner, lying on the dirt floor with some dirty blankets were two small, dirt smeared children, who were fast asleep. In another corner, lying on a raised pallet that was padded with some corrugated cardboard and an old mattress were three hound dogs. They made no disturbance, but merely raised their heads to look at me, and then put them down again to sleep some more.

The young man then steered me to a low doorway at the side of the room, saying that his wife was in there. I peered in, and in the light of a single dim light bulb I was able to see a large double bed, with some sheets and old blankets on it, and in it was a young woman who was obviously in labor and about to deliver. The problem with the room was that the ceiling was only about five feet high at its doorway, and then sloped downward as was common in a woodshed. I couldn't stand up next to the bed, and when I attempted to kneel at the bedside, I found that I wasn't tall enough to do anything effective.

This was not the first baby for this woman, and I felt that a delivery without any lacerations was possible, so I sat on the edge of the bed, and controlled the baby's birth so that when the baby was born the mother suffered no lacerations. The baby cried immediately, appeared to be wide awake, and seemed to be normal. After I made sure that the placenta was cleanly delivered, and none of it was missing, I gave the mother the usual injection of ergotrate, and left a few more doses in pill form for her. Then I had to write down some information, which would be needed to fill out a birth certificate, before I could leave.

Full daylight had arrived when I left the house, and as I crossed the yard I could confirm that it was indeed a large pile of garbage that I had walked over when I arrived. The house obviously had no indoor plumbing, so I looked about for an outhouse, but saw none. I was curious and looked again. Then I saw it, off to one side and slightly uphill. It didn't really look like a privy, so I went closer to have a better look. A shallow trench had been dug and at each end of it a pair of wooden fence posts had been set into the ground about three feet apart. A piece of 2x4 lumber had been nailed to them at about chair height, connecting the posts of each pair together. Then a long 2x4 ran the length of the trench from one crosspiece to the other. I assumed that it served as a crude toilet seat when the outhouse was used. For what there was of privacy in this situation, a single wire had been fastened up around the four posts at a height of about five feet from the ground, and a few opened-up burlap bags were hanging on it,------ an arrangement that certainly didn't allow for much privacy.

In the daylight I could see that there were other poor looking dwellings in the area in what appeared to be sort of a squatters' settlement. I assumed that the inhabitants had come there from the hills of Tennessee, lured by the higher wages supposedly available in Michigan. I visited there one more time later, to examine the patriarch of the settlement. I should have known better. It was a Saturday night, and everybody was thoroughly inebriated, even the little two and three year old children.

A Problem in Logistics

Long before I became a Deputy Medical Examiner I received an urgent call to come out to see one of my regular patients because of chest pain and shortness of breath. I had been treating her for hypertension and gross obesity, and although she had never demonstrated any signs or symptoms of heart failure, her complaint now sounded as if she were having severe angina pectoris or a coronary heart attack (coronary occlusion). She lived some three or four miles out of town in a farmhouse, which had been built many years before farmhouses had indoor plumbing, and the plumbing arrangement, which had later been added on, was anything but lavish.

It appeared that the first running water put into the house was piped into the kitchen, which was located in a back corner of the house. It included a sink and a drain. Bathing was still done in the kitchen in a tub, which was filled with water that was heated on the kitchen stove. It was then the custom of the times to bathe only about once a week.

When a flush toilet was added to the system later, it was necessary to place it strategically close to the water supply and sewage system, but it could, of course, not be installed in the kitchen. This resulted in the construction of an enclosed, narrow hallway, about three feet wide, and some twenty feet long, along the back, outside kitchen wall, with a door at one end and the toilet at the other. Actually this three-foot corridor had been "stolen" from the area of a glass-enclosed porch, which ran the full length of the back of the house. When the user was seated on the toilet he faced the door.

When I arrived at the house, the family members there were quite upset and told me that the patient had gone in to the "bathroom" and she was still "in there." I knew that it was fairly common that a patient having a heart attack would go to the toilet, and die sitting on the "throne," so I didn't hesitate, but went in right away. There, some twenty feet down that narrow hall, still seated on the toilet, was the patient, who weighed something over three hundred pounds. I got to her quickly, and found that she had indeed died while seated on the stool, but she had not fallen off. Her bulky body was wedged between the walls of that narrow hall and the back of the toilet.

After I explained that I thought she had died of a coronary heart attack, the family told me that they wanted the Pettit Funeral Home to handle all arrangements, so I called and explained to young Mr. Richard Pettit that there would be a logistical problem in getting the heavy, bulky body out of the toilet room. I offered to stay and help.

It was only about twenty minutes until the hearse arrived, with Richard and one helper, to pick up the body. Now to be faced was the problem of getting that huge body out of that long, narrow hall in a more or less dignified manner and without causing any damage. Dick Pettit and his helper seemed unfazed, and after carefully examining the problem, they went to work. First a partially folded canvas (a tarpaulin, I think) was spread out on the floor in front of the toilet. On top of it a soft blanket was placed. Then they went together, facing each other to the patient. Each grasped an arm and shoulder and pulled the body forward off of the stool, so that it stretched out, face down on that blanket. They covered it with another blanket. Then the two of them grasped the canvas, and each grasped one hand of the patient and pulled. The huge body slid smoothly along the hallway floor into the open, where, with additional help, they had no trouble placing it on their ambulance cart. I admired this maneuver. I thought it was a pretty neat and dignified solution to the problem.

The Tale of a Crazy Woman

Before I get into the story of this particular patient, I must explain that throughout my entire career I have never been keen on psychiatry as a separate part of medical practice. I was familiar with the principles and theories upon which psychiatry was based, but I didn't like the way those principles were often applied. I felt that the methods and details involved in treatment were mostly empty rituals and, at best, exercises in futility, and I was sure that to subject already anxious patients to formal psychiatric treatment served only to foster confusion, uncertainty, and fear. In many cases the cause of a patient's fear is quite apparent, and has a logical explanation. I believe that to subject such people to formal psychiatric treatment often creates mental problems where none existed before. My previous book, MOUNTAIN TROOPS AND MEDICS, includes the true story of my combat experiences in World War II, and in it I point out some very poor and perhaps harmful results produced by subjecting soldiers in our U.S. Army to unnecessary psychiatric treatment.

In my own practice I recognized that I often contributed to a patients' mental well being, not just by what I was honestly able to say, but more by what I had had been able to do for the patient. By always being honest and freely expressing my opinions and concerns about their health, by always telling them what I thought about their diagnosis, or perhaps by telling them that I was puzzled by their symptoms, and had not yet made a diagnosis, I achieved a reputation for honesty and directness. Eventually whatever I said, be it good news or bad, was believed completely, and I became an authority for medical information to most of my patients.

Physical disease generally has a psychological component, and no matter how small it may be, the mental well being of the patient should always be considered in any treatment program prescribed. Pure psychological illness does exist, however, and it is real. I have successfully treated such cases, and watched them recover, without calling upon a psychiatrist.

In my opinion there are two main basic underlying causes for pure psychological illness. They are fear and fatigue. Fear of the unknown seems to be the strongest, most chronic, and most potent of all fears, and I believe it is stronger than the fear of death or disability. Most patients, who are sick, harbor additional fears in their minds, which may affect how they feel. The "Combat Fatigue' or "Combat Exhaustion" which occurred in front line combat soldiers in my division in World War II is an excellent example of pure psychiatric illness in otherwise able bodied, healthy young men.

It seems obvious that treatment for such illness must be to first remove the underlying causes, that is, mitigate the patient's fear and allow for rest and sleep. A physician can do much toward this end, particularly in moderating fears about illness. In order to do this the physician must always be completely open and honest with the patient, explain the illness being treated and the reasons for any treatment prescribed. The more about their illness that patients can be taught, the better and more cooperative they will be. As years pass, the physician who practices in this way will develop a reputation for directness, honesty, and sympathetic care, and become ever more valuable in the service of medicine. In other words, then, what he says will be believed!

I was asked to see the patient in this story because she had a mental illness. She was being treated by a doctor who practiced in a neighboring town about ten miles from Eaton Rapids. The story that he gave me over the phone was that this was a woman in her mid-forties who was hallucinating and acting wild, and that the husband was asking to have her committed to a mental institution. In her present state it would be impossible to bring her in to my office without using force, so would I please see her at her home, and please, would I include in my report that the patient was in no condition to attend the hearing in Court. I understood the situation, and accepted the assignment reluctantly.

In those days in Michigan one could be completely crazy, and it could be obvious to everyone, but that person was not insane until a Court declared that the person was insane. Only after this legal truth had been established could the person be committed.

In the rural area, where I practiced, the courts required that two licensed physicians, after physically examining the patient within a specified time limit, must concur that the patient is indeed insane, and each must disclose the psychiatric diagnoses to the Court in the report of their findings. The Court must then hold a hearing during which the necessary declarations of insanity and commitment can be made. In this case the hearing was already scheduled for two or three days hence, and all of the paperwork had to be finished before the Court convened.

The patient lived on a farm several miles beyond our neighboring city, and there were several family members present when I arrived in the house, but I only remember the husband well. The woman herself, clad in a long nightgown and a robe that was badly wrinkled, had grossly unkempt hair and a "wild" look in her eye. It took some time for her husband to persuade her to come into the living room where I was to examine her. Then it took me a few minutes to get her to sit down and talk to me. I think that she recognized my medical bag, which I had placed next to me on the couch, and this seemed to reassure her that I meant her no harm.

It was obvious that she was having hallucinations. She was seeing people, both inside the house and outside, and she was seeing animals outside that weren't there. She was certain that all of them wanted to hurt her. Also, during our conversation she reassured me that a relative, who had just passed through the living room to leave the house, was Jesus Christ.

Delusions and hallucinations are present in major psychiatric illnesses, the names of which have changed as years have passed. In those days we were calling this one Dementia Praecox, and the courts seemed to understand what it meant.

When the patient had gained enough confidence in me to be able to talk more or less freely, I began to take a real health history. Several points stood out. For several months she had had spells of severe anxiety, which came and went. She had intermittent abdominal bloating severe enough to make her very uncomfortable. Recurrent headaches, and swelling of her hands and feet were present much of the time. There were skipped menstrual periods, which made her exceptionally fearful because she did not want to be pregnant, and finally there were the numerous hot flushes, which were occurring day and night. To me this added up to menopausal syndrome, and I said so. Further inquiry indicated that she had apparently never received any treatment for it.

So I suggested to the patient and her husband that we try to treat her symptoms by giving her a "hormone shot." I explained that this often cleared up many of the symptoms that she had been having, but I was careful not to add my thought that perhaps she wasn't "insane," and that perhaps all of her symptoms could be due to menopause. The patient and her husband agreed, and I gave her an intramuscular injection of estrogen in oil, such as I was giving regularly to other women in menopause. In this form the hormone would be slowly absorbed, and would treat the symptoms for about three weeks. I asked the husband to let me know by phone if it did any good.

The next day I wrote up my findings for the Court, but only up to the point of certifying that the patient was not in condition to appear at the hearing. That evening I received a phone call from the husband who said that he was amazed at the change in his wife. She seemed to be her old self again. She acted sensibly again, and was no longer any trouble to herself or her family. He no longer wanted to commit her. With the court hearing only thirty-six hours away, what should he do?

I considered his question, and then told him that I could not change the report of my visit and my examination to the court, but I would omit the statement that the patient would not be able to appear in Court. I would add that I thought much of her problem was due to menopause, and that I had initiated treatment for menopausal symptoms. I suggested that the patient herself go to the court hearing in person to demonstrate that she was acting well.

I also told her husband that the effect of the shot I had given her should last for three to four weeks, and that when the effect seemed to be wearing off she could get more shots as needed from her own doctor.

Then I wrote to her doctor immediately, explaining what I had done. I know that this lady was not committed as the result of that hearing, and that she went back to her own doctor for treatment for several years afterward.

CHAPTER XXI

OFFICE STORIES

From a patient's viewpoint there is little humor in a physician's office, and whenever humorous situations do occur, the information is usually shared only by the office staff. Patients hardly ever learn about it.

My office had a large waiting room, which was shared by all of the other doctors in our medical group, and people seemed to enjoy its social atmosphere to the extent that many regularly came in for their medical appointment well ahead of time. There were a few ladies who arrived for their appointment as much as three hours early, and occasionally one would show up in our waiting room with no appointment and no intention of seeing a doctor at all. This group included one or two ladies who made it a point to attend almost every funeral in town.

Our waiting room didn't really seem like a doctors' waiting room, because it was usually crowded with people, and there was usually much conversation. I'm sure that much news, dirt and gossip was exchanged. The stories that follow here in this section are related to office practice more than less. Some appear here because I forgot to include them somewhere else, or I didn't know where else to put them.

Dermatology to the Rescue

One of my very early patients was a woman in her late-twenties. She had multiple complaints, but her main one was that she had low abdominal pain, and her menstrual periods were not regular. They were prolonged, often with painful cramping. The first time I examined her I easily put her into my patient category classification as one of the "unwashed." She appeared to be one of those women who thought a constant vaginal discharge was normal. In spite of her complaints I could find no evidence of a major problem. She obviously had a mild, chronic pelvic infection, which, in those days, was difficult, if not impossible, to cure. Before antibiotics became available, all we had to offer were douches designed to sterilize the vagina, and heat applications to treat the internal pelvic organs. Often the infection would clear up, but it was the patient's own defenses (immune system) which accomplished the cure. If infection had been long-standing with persistent symptoms, we knew that scar tissue and adhesions had formed in the pelvis, and recommended surgical excision of the chronically infected organs when necessary to relieve the pain.

During the examination of this patient I made and examined vaginal smears, and satisfied myself that there were no gonococci present. Then I personally instructed the patient in how to douche, and prescribed a course of a sulfonamide (sulfa drug). Penecillin was available in those days, but only in the injectable form, that we normally administered every three hours to patients who were hospitalized.

When this woman returned some three weeks later, I was most pleased to see that she had improved greatly. The improvement did not last however, and I saw her several more times. I prescribed special douching solutions, more heat applications and repeat courses of sulfonamide drugs. It was during that series of visits that I noted that she did not appear to be bathing, or laundering her underclothing. It had come to the point where I was seeing the same menstrual blood stains on her slip during several consecutive visits. My admonishments about cleanliness and personal hygiene did not seem to be producing any results. I tried the hygiene lecture approach several times, and explained to her that the least she could do was wash her underpants every day to keep the crotch from rubbing more germs up into her vagina.

The next time she visited I noted that she was wearing clean, new panties of the kind that were made of rayon, which could be bought at the local dime store for about twenty five cents. Her complaints however were still the same. During her next few visits I noted that she always wore brand new, clean underpants, and I got her to admit that she wore them every day without laundering until the day of her next doctor appointment. It was then that she donned a newly purchased pair in which to come to my office. I was scratching my head to try to find a way to get her to change her habits.

Then one day she appeared in my office with a new complaint. She itched, and as near as I could tell, she had a mild rash on her abdomen, back and a little on her extremities. I knew that she had a bathtub at home, so saw this as an opportunity. I quickly wrote out a prescription for Sergeants Dog Soap, which I knew was especially mild and non-irritating, because dogs are known to have sensitive skin. The prescription, written in Latin read: ***Saponis Sargenti – Bar 1.*** Instructions were: **Once daily, in the bathtub, wet the body all over. Rub the medicine all over entire body. Allow to remain for five minutes. Then rinse thoroughly.**

My patient had gone immediately across the street to the drug store and Glyn Shimmin, the owner and pharmacist, called me right away, wanting to know if I was in my right mind. I assured him that I was, and told him to wrap or box the soap bar without any of the original wrappings, and to put his prescription label on it. Furthermore he must do the same whenever she returned for refills.

This did the trick. I did not see the patient again for several months, and thought that perhaps she was mad at me for the dog soap prescription. However, I did see her a few more times before she moved away from our area. She was bathed and all of her clothing was clean. She reported that she enjoyed taking bubble baths. I never did tell her about the dog soap, but I was a truly amazed that a mild skin rash, for which I had not even made a diagnosis, and my treatment of it had wrought such an amazing change in this young woman's behavior.

Cookies Anyone?

It happens in many physicians' offices. A number of the motherly type women patients bring treats in to the office for their doctor and the office personnel. Usually it is something edible, and home made, such as cookies, cake, doughnuts, fudge and other candies. One of the regulars who brought us something to eat almost every time she came in was an elderly widow who lived out of town on a farm. Because it is not her name, I shall refer to her as Sophie. She was a good-hearted soul. She dressed in clothing that I would classify as a bit grimy, but she had no noticeable body odor. What struck almost everyone who met her for the first time were her hands. They were always dirty, with black muck from the garden under her fingernails. Sophie's treats were often baked goods, and the mental image of Sophie's hands kneading the dough, or even handling the cookies, was enough to turn most of the people who knew her away from her treats. Actually what she brought in wasn't bad. I ate some of her cookies from time to time, and there were no untoward consequences.

The other half of this story is that there were a number of women who were first class cooks and bakers. Whenever something from one of these people appeared in the back room at the office, whatever it was would disappear fast. Many times I noticed a box or a dish of these super treats on the counter, but I was rushed, very busy, and couldn't take time to eat then. By the time I could get back, the goodies were usually gone. I found a way to solve this problem. As I walked past the treats on the counter I would say in a loud voice,

"These cookies (or whatever) that Sophie brought in certainly look good."

Invariably there would be some left for me at the end of office hours.

An Imagined Catastrophe

My patient was a well-known, well-liked teacher in the Eaton Rapids Public Schools, who was nearing retirement age. She had been in good health all of her life, but in recent years had gradually gained weight until the extra weight had become a health problem. In addition to carrying extra, unneeded weight, she had developed some hypertension for which I had prescribed diet and medication. It was obvious that she had a hard time sticking to the diet, but her blood pressure levels remained reasonable. She had also become a worrier, and on each visit to my office she would tell me about the terrible things happening to people with high blood pressure who were also overweight. However, in her demeanor, dress and grooming, she was a refined, knowledgeable, old maid schoolteacher.

One day in the middle of a week my office received a call from Miss ______ who was at school. The receptionist reported to me that she sounded upset and agitated, but wouldn't say exactly what the trouble was, so she told her to come in right away. Miss ______ said that she had to finish out the school day. So the arrangement was changed to have her come in as soon as she could, and I would see her quickly.

She arrived later that afternoon, and I happened to observe her arrival. She had a "wild" expression on her face, and her face was very red. She was breathing hard, and appeared agitated. My nurse led her into an examining room immediately, and I soon followed. Her pupils were large, her face was very flushed, and she was sweating.

"Oh doctor," she almost shouted, "something terrible is happening to me. I've been worried sick all day."

"What is the trouble?" I asked

"This morning" she continued, "when I went to the toilet my stool sank right to the bottom of the bowl, instead of floating like it usually does!!!"

I didn't want to laugh in front of the patient, but under the circumstances this statement struck me as being so funny that I knew I wouldn't be able to maintain my usual earnest, down-to-business facial expression. I quickly excused myself and left the room.

After gaining my composure I went back into the room. My patient looked much better, and no longer seemed agitated. I discussed in some detail the specific gravity of fecal material, and why some floated and some didn't. This was all that was needed, and when Miss ______ left my office her blood pressure was again normal, her face was no longer flushed, and she seemed like a different person.

Success Through Procrastination

This case began while I still had my office in Stimson Hospital. The sixteen-year-old girl came in to see me because she had pain in her lower abdomen and bleeding from the vagina of more that twenty-four hour's duration. She seemed to me to be larger and more developed than most girls of her age, and except for the vaginal bleeding, she appeared to be healthy. Prior to this visit I had known her, and I knew that she had a reputation of being a bit "wild."

It was difficult to obtain the history of her present illness from her because she seemed reluctant to tell me the whole story, but after some careful questioning in detail, it all came out. She had missed several menstrual periods. She thought she was pregnant, and had put potassium permanganate into her vagina in the hope of creating a miscarriage. Potassium permanganate was readily and widely available because in those days various strength solutions of it were frequently used to soak fungus infections, such as athlete's foot, in order to produce a cure. It acted as a strong oxidation agent, much as a strong bleaching solution does, but it also stained everything that it touched a dirty brown color. At the beginning nothing had happened. Then after some hours she began to spot a little blood from the vagina. The next day the bleeding became heavier, she became alarmed, and came to the office to see me.

When I started to examine her, I could feel the enlarged uterus in her abdomen, and estimated that it represented a pregnancy that was about four months along. I should perhaps have heard a fetal heart but I didn't, and surmised that it was either too early to hear it, or that the fetus was dead. The perineal pad she was wearing was well soaked with blood, so I decided to take her upstairs into surgery, where I could apply more extensive treatment if needed, and examine her vagina and uterine cervix under sterile conditions.

Using a vaginal speculum to hold the vagina open, I removed several large blood clots and found that there were crystals of potassium permanganate still present in the upper vagina and around the cervix. This made me wonder if someone else had placed it there for her, perhaps using a funnel of some kind, because the lower vagina seemed not to be injured, only stained brown as some of the chemical flowed out with the blood. I did not pursue this, however, because it was important that the girl must trust me and follow my instructions in order to make a good recovery from this insult. I irrigated the vagina with a large amount of plain sterile water until I thought that all of the chemical had been washed out. During this process I observed that the exterior of the cervix had been severely chemically burned, and the entire upper vault of the vagina, around its 360-degree circumference, had likewise been burned. The entire surface area of the upper two inches of the vagina was badly damaged, and there was still a considerable amount of bleeding, so I placed gauze packing against the damaged area, and left it there for several hours. Later, when I removed it, the upper vagina and cervix looked like a huge black hole, but the bleeding had stopped, giving way to a little oozing of serum. The immediate crisis had been overcome, and I let the girl go home with specific instructions not to put anything at all into her vagina, and gave her a time to return to my office to check on her progress.

Although I thought that the fetus had already died, I chose to let the patient continue regular prenatal visits to my office, at least until I could be sure. On the first visit back the upper vagina looked much better. Granulation tissue (the precursor of scar tissue) was already beginning to form. I could hear no fetal heart tones, and I thought that perhaps the uterus had become a bit smaller. A month later I was sure that the uterus was smaller, and I was certain that the fetus had died. The upper vagina had continued to heal, and now I could identify the opening of the cervix, but there was still a large raw area, which I thought would take a long time to heal.

Now we faced the problem of what to do about the uterine contents. I did a lot of research and reading about this subject, and found recommendations to empty the uterus by doing dilatation (of the cervix) and curettage, and recommendations to operate and empty the uterus as in a caesarian section. I liked the conservative recommendations better. They essentially advised to leave the uterus alone, and in time the dead fetal tissues would be either reabsorbed or passed out with the first several menstrual periods when they resumed. I was very leery of doing a curettage of a uterus, especially one connected with pregnancy, because of the large amount of bleeding it might cause, and the increased possibility of severely damaging or perforating the uterus.

So I kept the patient happy and bought time by telling her that if we treated her as if she were still pregnant, she would go into labor and pass the remains of the dead fetus on her due date. She kept her prenatal appointments, and I was "off the hook" when, the day after her due date, she began to cramp, bleed a little. And passed some scraps of long-dead tissue. After that, without further treatment she began having regular menstrual periods that were quite normal.

Before I dismissed her from my care, I did a last pelvic examination in my office, and found that the upper vagina had healed, but there was a wide, heavy, circular band of scar tissue surrounding the cervical canal in the upper vagina. I was certain that this "donut of scar" could never be dilated sufficiently to allow a vaginal delivery. I knew that the cervix was open because I could identify the opening, and she was having regular periods with normal blood flow. Therefore I told her that I thought that she could still become pregnant, but that she could never have a vaginal delivery, because the opening could not be stretched enough to allow it.

The happy ending here is that this girl later got married, and had two lovely, normal children. I took care of her pregnancies, and did the caesarian sections.

Tattoo Tale No. 1

Throughout the years I saw many patients with tattoos in various places on their bodies, and some of them gave rise to humorous situations. Not funny however was the case of a relatively young man who had prominent, decorative tattoos on both forearms, and who was finally employed in a position in which he wore a long-sleeved shirt, tie, and jacket. This costume hid his tattoos admirably well, but from time to time he was required to shed the jacket and roll up his shirtsleeves. This allowed his tattoos to be out in plain sight of everyone nearby, and because at this time in his life he had become ashamed of the tattoos, he consulted me about having them removed.

Because tattoos are created by injecting indelible pigments into the actual skin tissue with a needle, I knew of no way that a tattoo could be removed except by excising the area of skin involved. In my opinion tattooing was a dubious and dangerous practice because of the unknown infectious materials, which might be included in the pigments. I had seen two or three cases in which a person had tried to hide a tattoo by tattooing over it with skin-colored pigments, and the results were very poor. It is difficult to exactly match skin color, and impossible to allow for changes in normal skin color as in summer sun tanning versus winter pallor. I had to tell this patient that the only sure way to remove his tattoos was to excise the skin in which they were contained. They were so large that to excise the whole tattoo in this manner would leave a skin defect so large that it would not be possible to close it, without covering it with a skin graft, and that the skin of the graft would forever look different than the normal surrounding skin. I recommended removing the skin in stages, beginning with the removal of an ellipse of skin through the middle of the tattoo, undermining the skin edges enough to be able to slide them together, and closing the defect with stitches. After this wound was well healed, the remaining skin would be stretched, and would attenuate itself about the forearm. When this process was complete, and the skin remaining had loosened up a bit, a second removal of an elliptical piece of skin, which included the scar from the first operation, could be done. If enough time could be allowed between each procedure to allow the remaining skin around the forearm to loosen up well, the operation could be repeated until the tattoos were gone.

The patient elected to do this, and I repeated the operation four or five times over a period of several years. The tattoos were finally gone, leaving a linear scar, lengthwise on each forearm.

Tattoo Tale No. 2

A mother with two daughters came in to the office to see me. The daughters were aged 14 and 16 years. The 16 year old had a "swollen belly", and was presumed to be pregnant. Sure enough, when I had her lie down on the table to examine her abdomen, it protruded noticeably. When we got it undraped down to the bare skin, I was suddenly amused by the prominent tattoo, in letters about one inch high, running across the abdomen from side to side, which read, "MADE IN AMERICA".

It was easy to confirm the diagnosis because when I listened I could easily rear the strong, steady fetal heart. After completing an initial pre-natal visit, the mother asked if I would prescribe birth control pills for her 14-year-old daughter. After hearing about all of the loose living which was going on in that family, I agreed that it would be a good idea, and supplied her with a prescription for two months, in order to give her time to contact the County Social Services Department for further care.

Tattoo Tale No. 3

This patient was a middle aged married woman who had a reputation about town for "wild living." She was known to smoke a lot, imbibe alcohol frequently, and had an unusually large vocabulary of profanity. When she wanted to, she could cut loose with a string of it that would make most of the people blush. She came to see me in my office in the Stimson Hospital building one afternoon, claiming that during the past night she had been "beaten up" by her husband.

This alerted me to the fact that she might want to press charges to the law against her husband, so I needed to make a through examination, and make a good written record of her actual physical injuries. I did a reasonably thorough examination and found only bruises and skin abrasions. There was no evidence of injury anywhere deep inside the body

When I examined the bruises and abrasions on her legs I was confronted with a prominent, large tattoo on the inside of the left thigh. In letters about two inches high was tattooed the word, "DICK", and running from it, pointing up toward her vagina was an ornate arrow.

Her problem the night before began with she and her husband in bed, possibly not completely sober. When her husband saw the tattoo he got mad, and promptly beat her up.

CHAPTER XXII

EMERGENCY ROOM STORIES

Except for events in actual front line combat in World War II, the most exciting medical events that happened to me during my career occurred in the emergency room. My first experiences with emergencies occurred when I was an intern at Sparrow Hospital in Lansing. Next came the emergencies of the battlefield. Later my involvement with emergency medicine grew with the evolvement of emergency services in Eaton Rapids. For a number of my early years in practice I was a member of the American Academy of Family Practice, but when the American College of Emergency Physicians was organized in Lansing, I became a charter member. Soon afterward I had become so involved with surgery and emergencies that I dropped out of the family practice group. When the American College of Emergency Physicians (ACEP) developed the American Board of Emergency Physicians for the purpose of certifying properly trained, Board Certified Emergency Physicians, I took and passed the first certifying examination given by this board. I was over sixty years old then, and might possibly have been the oldest one to take the exam.

Here are some of the "adventures" in emergencies in which I was involved during my career.

Sudden Anaphylaxis

When my office was in Stimson Hospital, and my large examining room did double duty as an emergency room, there occurred some exciting times. I remember giving a young woman an injection of penecillin during office hours. In a few minutes she collapsed to the floor in a manner typical of anaphylactic shock. She was pale and pasty in appearance, unconscious, obviously short of breath, and had copious diarrhea. She had a very feeble pulse, but there was no time to check the blood pressure. Fortunately this happened in that pseudo-emergency room, and injectable epinephrine (Adrenalin) was immediately at hand. I injected a large dose into her immediately, and signs of improvement quickly appeared. I breathed a sigh of relief, and after the administration of some other medicines, admitted her to the hospital. This happened in the days before a drug to neutralize penecillin in the body was available, so it was necessary to keep close watch over her, which we did for two or three days. Her recovery was complete, and she went home with the dire warning to avoid penecillin, or anything the might have penecillin in it.

Allergic sensitivity such as this develops in some individuals, but it only develops after the individual has been previously exposed to the offending substance, and after a critical period of time after the exposure has elapsed. There is no reaction to the initial exposure, and then, after the appropriate interval of time has gone by, subsequent exposures will trigger these reactions. In the case of penecillin, many people were showing allergic reactions to it with no history of ever having had penecillin previously. We blamed this on milk and dairy products, because at the time it was common in veterinary medicine to treat mastitis and inflammation in the udders of milk cows by placing inserts containing penecillin into the milk ducts. Enough traces of penecillin remained in the milk, which was distributed for public consumption, to cause a penecillin sensitivity to develop in some people. Penecillin was widely known to cause allergic reactions and anaphylaxis. Many practicing physicians carried with them a nagging dread that something like this would happen to one of their patients. Indeed, the case of anaphylaxis I have just described occurred not long after we had learned that a well-known Lansing doctor had given his own son an injection of penecillin, only to have him die of anaphylactic shock before his very eyes.

Chinese Water Torture

Another case that sticks in my memory occurred in that same room late one evening at a time when I was on emergency duty. The patient was a middle-aged woman who had been involved in some kind of a quarrel at home. She was brought in by ambulance, and I had the attendants place her on the examining table. A family member was present and reported that the woman had "passed out" during the argument at home, and had been unconscious ever since. It took only a moment for me to realize that she was not unconscious. Although her eyes were closed, the eyelids were fluttering and from time to time she squeezed them tightly together. When I tried to open one eye by gently lifting the lid, she resisted. The eyelids of dead and unconscious people never resist when one is raised to examine the pupil. This patient was a good actress, and was able to endure some moderately painful test stimuli without moving. I didn't want to increase the strength of the stimuli for fear of damaging her flesh, so I decided to try the Chinese Water Torture. We hooked up a large enema can filled with plain water with a rubber hose ending in an eye dropper, then dripped the water, one drop at a time, onto her face and nose. Fifteen or twenty drops caused her head to move, but no other change occurred. The water drops followed her nose wherever it moved. There was more movement, but still the water drops kept dripping on her nose. This game had gone on for about five minutes when the patient abruptly sat up, jumped spryly down from the table and said for all present to hear,

"This is a hell of a way to treat a sick person!"

Then she flounced out of the room and out of the building. I don't remember ever seeing her again.

Severe Burns

Daytime emergencies were also cared for. I remember a two-year-old girl, who arrived in her mother's arms in the middle of the morning, with severe second-degree burns over a large area of her body. Her mother had been doing the family laundry, and had just taken a tub full of boiling water off of the stove and placed it on the floor. The child had fallen into it, but luckily there was a second tub of cold water nearby, and the mother snatched the girl out of the hot tub and put her into the cold one. This act probably saved that child's life. Fortunately the face, neck, arms and legs below the knees were not burned, but the entire torso, buttocks and most of the thighs had huge blisters on them. I did not see anything that looked like third degree burns, but all of these areas certainly had severe second-degree burns.

During the recent War, I had seen and treated a little girl at the front when I was a Battalion Surgeon in the mountain infantry in Italy. I didn't have much to work with there, so I covered the burns with a substantial occlusive dressing, and had the family leave it in place for 10 days. When they returned the bandage was still intact, but dripping out from under the edges was what looked like pure pus, and it was incredibly foul smelling. When I took that bandage off I was most gratified to see clean, new, pink skin with no sign of scarring anywhere. Although the burns in my present case were more extensive I decided to treat them in the same way. I believed that they would heal in the same way as the as the burns of the child in Italy had healed. However, I didn't quite trust the home care that this girl would receive, so after applying the occlusive dressings, I put her into a plaster body cast, which included the chest, torso and thighs. I even incorporated a wooden handle into the plaster between the thighs, so that the caregivers would have a convenient handle to aid in carrying the child. I also increased the cover-up time to two weeks, and when the time came to remove the cast, I was again faced with the same smelly situation that I had seen in Italy. The cast was still intact but appeared battered and was beginning to crumble in places. The stench was terrible. However, when I removed the cast and the dressings, the skin underneath looked beautiful. This little girl also grew up without any scarring from the burn!

Lacerated Ear

One day a father brought his seven or eight-year-old son in with the story that he, the father, had been dragging a disk (farm implement) over some local muck land behind a tractor, and the boy was riding with him. During a turn in the field the boy fell off and was partially run over by the disk. Eaton County muck is possibly the blackest on Earth, and this boy was covered with it from head to foot. The most obvious injury he had sustained was to his right ear, which had been almost severed from his head. Fortunately it had not been completely severed, because it would then have probably been lost forever in the muck in the field.

Cleanup was in order. First I cleaned up the face, head, and area about the ear with liquid soap and water, and applied a temporary bandage. Next the nurses gave him a tub bath. Then we took him back to our "emergency room" and I examined him thoroughly. Except for some skin scrapes and minor bruises, there were no signs of other serious injury. The dangling ear was the main problem. Using local anesthesia, I cleaned it and examined it carefully. The only connection that the ear had with the rest of the head was a skin bridge about one inch wide behind the ear. The ear cartilage had been completely severed, leaving only the cartilaginous part of the external ear canal behind. I was skeptical that the ear could survive re-attachment, but I did put it back in place using the stitching technique that I have previously described, in which no suture material remains in the wound site after all of the stitches have been removed. I used very fine, thin, non-absorbable suture material. Then with a dressing applied, and the re-attached ear gently splinted against the boy's head, I admitted him to the hospital. We treated the ear with ice packs in order to lower the metabolism in the severed part, so that it could survive without as much oxygen as it would otherwise need. As best I can remember, the antibiotic I prescribed was a combination of penecillin and streptomycin. The boy did not develop a fever, and the ear did not die. Sutures were removed early and by the fifth day the boy was discharged from the hospital with about half of them still in place. The next week in the office I removed all of the rest of the stitches, and the ear still looked good. As I recall, although I asked to see him again, the family never brought him back to me, and I never saw or heard from them again. This boy came from a poor, dirt farmer family that lived from hand to mouth. I am certain that I was not paid for my services in this case, nor was the hospital. All I had was a good feeling, knowing that I had saved the boy's ear and prevented an ugly deformity which only expensive, reconstructive, plastic surgery might fix later.

Death of a Child

I still think occasionally about one ugly human tragedy connected with that room in Stimson Hospital, which occurred during my shift on call. That morning a parent carried in the body of a little girl, about two years old. She had been accidentally shot by a sibling who was not much older. The family lived in a trailer home in a rural area, and the sibling had found a loaded shotgun in a closet, had taken it out and was apparently playing with it when it discharged, killing the little sister instantly. There was nothing to do to help the dead child, but much to do to ease this tragedy for the child's parents and grandparents. The entire scene at the hospital took only a few minutes, but I still remember it vividly.

Endotracheal Intubation

One of the most important new skills I developed during my career in medicine was that of endotracheal intubation, in which a "breathing tube" is placed between the patient's vocal cords into the upper trachea (windpipe), and a doughnut shaped balloon encircling the tube near its lower end is inflated to create a tight seal between the tube and the trachea. Once in place such a tube guarantees an open airway, which can be used for artificial respiration and the administration of oxygen, as well as for the administration of certain anesthetic agents.

Because of gagging, choking and spasm of the vocal cords it is practically impossible to insert such a tube into a conscious person's trachea, and I believe that to attempt such a thing borders on cruelty. In anesthesia the usual procedure is to render the patient unconscious with an intravenous anesthetic agent, then completely paralyze him with succinylcholine or curare, which paralyzes every muscle in the body including those which are needed for breathing, and those that control the vocal cords. Because only three or four minutes without breathing will cause brain damage, it becomes urgent to quickly insert the endotracheal tube and, through it, breathe for the patient. This is not always easily done.

In obese people, and people with short necks, a maximum extension of the neck will not allow direct vision of the vocal cords, and the anesthetist may need to insert the tube blindly. This can be and often is done, but it is very difficult unless the person passing the tube is completely familiar with the normal anatomy of the throat and airway and is well practiced in the maneuver. The immediate urgency caused by the fact that the patient is not breathing can also be a detriment to a smooth passage of the tube.

By giving the anesthetist more complete control over the patient's vital functions, endotracheal intubation changed the practice of anesthesia when it became possible to completely paralyze all muscles and breathe for the patient. Paralyzing the abdominal muscles removed almost all of the resistance encountered by the surgeon during abdominal operations, allowed for shorter incisions, and avoided overdosing with anesthetic drugs and the sometimes long time required for the patient's body to excrete them.

Learning to pass an endotracheal tube was not easy for me. Dr. Sherman of our group was the first to master the procedure, and with him standing at my elbow I was able to pass a tube a few times. Some of these passages that I did were blindly done when they should have been done after visualization of the vocal cords, but I often couldn't see them even when I thought that I had the laryngoscope properly placed.

Then one summer afternoon an ambulance brought a little old lady in to our emergency room with the story that she had been found in a cornfield with her throat cut. She had been missing all day. She had apparently gone out into the field with a long butcher knife, and had cut her own throat. She had partially severed the trachea (windpipe), and was passing air in and out through the incision. She had cut several muscles, but the main arteries, veins and nerves in the neck had not been injured. Accurate surgical repair was indicated, and this time it became my lot to be the anesthetist. Intubation was indicated in order to keep control of the airway, and if the balloon cuff of the endotracheal tube could be placed below the opening in it, the trachea could be repaired more easily over the tube.

With the patient on the operating table, and the overhead operating light focused on her neck, I administered enough sodium pentothal to render her unconscious, then succinylcholine to relax all muscles. When I slipped the laryngoscope blade in I was startled to see the entire anatomy clearly. The overhead light passed through the hole in the trachea and clearly backlighted the vocal cords. The tube went in under my direct vision, and the surgeon could tell me how far down it had to go.

The repair was successful, and a week later the patient went home. I never saw this patient again, but ever after this incident I have been much more confident in passing endotracheal tubes, and have been very successful in doing it.

The Tale of Mister Lucky

Mister Lucky was not the patient's name, but is a name that I mentally pinned on him the morning after I did his extensive emergency surgery. I have long since forgotten his real name, but in my mind today he is still Mr. Lucky.

Our acquaintance grew out of a series of office visits during which he repeatedly complained about low back pain. He claimed to have injured himself while working at one of the General Motors Plants (either Oldsmobile or Fisher Body) in Lansing, and he stated repeatedly that the pain was too severe to let him do any work. After several such visits I had done a reasonably complete investigation of his complaint, including x-rays and mobility tests, and all of my investigative effort turned up nothing but normal results. I had to tell him that I couldn't find any physical reason for his pain, but privately I thought that he was probably "goldbricking," which is an old military expression with which I was very familiar. I offered some advice and gave him a pep talk, and he finally agreed to try to return to work, with the reservation that he needed several more weeks of rest and recuperation. In the end I signed the insurance papers and a "return to work" discharge for him.

Three weeks later I received a phone call from the General Motors Plant doctor. He said he was turning down the "return to work" status that I had recommended. From the discussion between us I surmised that he agreed with my findings and recommendations, but the higher up executives at General Motors were leery of a possible lawsuit and wanted the man put back on sick leave. We doctors were in no position to argue with that!

So I went through the whole thing with him again: office visits, insurance papers, sick leave and compensation papers, my discharge permission to return to work, and the subsequent veto by General Motors Management.

Before this problem with his back arose I had already known Mr. Lucky for some time, and had, in the past, delivered a child for him. I don't remember his wife's name, but I do remember her appearance very well. Her chronic haggard, woe-be-gone expression seemed always to reflect the trying conditions under which she lived. When I examined her for her pregnancy, I found that she had an enlarged heart and the typical heart murmurs of mitral stenosis and insufficiency, which are caused by heart valve damage almost always due to rheumatic fever. She did not yet have obvious heart failure, but I felt sure that she had lived with this problem since childhood. She was now in her third decade of life, and in those days it was common for people with this kind of heart disease to die from progressive heart failure at a young age. Rarely did any of them live beyond their 45th birthday. I felt sorry for her, not only for that, but also for the conditions under which she lived at home, with several small children and a meager family income. The family lived far out of town where she helped make ends meet by raising chickens and tending a vegetable garden. Mr. Lucky also raised coonhounds, but not as a business. He was, himself, an avid raccoon hunter.

One afternoon in the summer three of my obstetrical patients were in labor at one time, and I made several trips across the street from my office to check on them. When office hours ended, two of the labors were well advanced, and I felt it necessary to stay at the hospital in order to be sure to be there when I was needed. I called my wife to tell her that I wouldn't be home for dinner, but because at that time we had a live-in baby-sitter who could feed the children, she should meet me across the street from the hospital obstetrical wing at the Dairy Queen, which was a fast-food business specializing in "soft" ice cream and a variety of sandwiches.

She agreed, and we were soon sitting in her car eating our supper in the parking area. This happened to be the year of the trampoline craze. Large trampolines were appearing all over, and people of all ages paid by the minute to jump up and down on them.

There was one next to this Dairy Queen, and I soon recognized the man who was jumping up and down on it. He was Mr. Lucky! We watched as he jumped high in the air again and again. He turned somersaults, assumed various positions in the air, landed on his buttocks often and on his back occasionally, always returning expertly to his upright position on his feet.

"See that man on the trampoline?" I said to my wife.

"Yes," she replied.

"He's one of my patients. He can't work because he has a bad back. I've been sending reports to General Motors about his condition for several months now. I thought he was faking from the beginning, and this demonstration seems to prove it."

Just then a door at the hospital across the street opened and the obstetrical nurse appeared waving a towel, which was the signal that I was needed right away. So my wife drove home, and I ran across the street to deliver the first of three babies that came into the world that night.

The summer and fall passed, and as we were entering the Christmas season, we scheduled the annual office Christmas dinner for the Eaton

Rapids Medical Clinic for the evening of the second Saturday before Christmas. This seemed a bit early at the time but we were glad to have it over and finished before the more serious Christmas festivities began. The turkey and other foods were paid for by the clinic, but Effie Fuller made all of the arrangements and did everything else for the party with help from some of the other employees of the clinic,

This year we rented a hall downtown. The table decorations and the food were great, and the exchange of token gifts was hilarious. Then came the call from the hospital. The ambulance was bringing in an injured man. I was the doctor "on call," so I left immediately headed for the hospital.

When the EMTs (Emergency Medical Technicians) wheeled the patient in, I recognized him right away. He was Mr. Lucky, and he was in severe pain. His story was quickly told.

It was common practice for raccoon hunts to be held after dark at night, and he had gone out with some of his hounds on such a "coon hunt." Faced by a barbed wire fence, made up of individual single strands fastened to heavy steel fence posts, he decided to climb over it. He had climbed up to stand on the top strand of barbed wire, with one foot on each side of a steel post, when the wire snapped and he was immediately impaled on the post.

We cut his blue jeans and his underwear off and I examined the wound. The post had struck the right side of his scrotum, ripped it open, then penetrated upward into the abdominal cavity. There was no sign of the testicle to be seen, so I had to assume that it had been pushed up into the abdomen. I was sure that there was other injury up there, which would lead to serious complications unless treated immediately. He was in dire need of a life-saving surgical exploration of his abdominal cavity. So I ordered the standard preoperative injections, which would also relieve much of the pain. I called the still ongoing Christmas party, and asked the surgical team to come in for the emergency operation.

Common sense required that the abdomen had to be opened and thoroughly explored for damage, and all damage had to be repaired promptly. Secondly the wound in the abdominal wall had to be repaired, and lastly the spermatic cord and testicle must be preserved, if possible, and replaced in the scrotum, which also had to be repaired.

Dr. Sherman gave the anesthesia, which involved intubation, artificial respiration, and muscle relaxants. I don't remember now who the assistant surgeon was, or who the nurses were. There must have been at least two of them. I made a right-sided, vertical incision in the abdomen. It was long, but I could easily lengthen it more if needed. When I opened the peritoneum, the innermost layer of the abdominal wall, the first thing I recognized was the patient's testicle, lying neatly next to the gall bladder up under the liver. It did not seem to be damaged, nor did the liver or the gallbladder show any signs of damage. I found a small patch of blue denim nearby, which the fence post had obviously punched out of the blue jeans as it passed through them. Of course I removed it, because to leave it behind would be to guarantee the development of infection and peritonitis. Next I carefully examined the spermatic cord in which lies the vas deferens, the tube that carries sperm away from the testicle, and the arteries and veins that supply the testicle and its appendages with blood flow. There seemed to be very little damage here, and nothing that I thought could be serious, so I carefully traced and followed the cord to the level where its blood supply comes off of the pelvic circulation, then shoved the testis back down the same path it had traveled to get into the abdomen. It fell nicely into the scrotum. Now I carefully examined all of the organs along this path: stomach, bile ducts, pancreas, duodenum, small bowel, colon, kidney, and I found no evidence of any severe damage. Some minor bruising was all there was!

The next step in the operation was to close the abdominal incision that I had made. After a careful lavage of the abdominal cavity with a physiological saline solution in order to wash away and dilute any bacteria which might be present, I did a routine closure, but took the precaution of inserting a soft rubber drain through the abdominal wall, so that if pus were to develop anywhere along the path that the steel fence post had taken inside of the abdomen, it would show up through the drain immediately. With such a drain in place, post-operative infection can be detected early, and can be cleared up by shortening the drain in small increments to allow the drain track to close up slowly from the inside out.

Now we knew that there had to be some damage to the inguinal canal, which is the passageway through which the testicle migrates during embryonic development in order to assume its proper place in the scrotum. To evaluate this I made a second incision, exactly like I would have made had I been repairing an inguinal hernia. Again I was surprised by the small amount of damage present. The external and internal inguinal rings were stretched and slightly torn, but the deep epigastric vessels on the backside of the canal seemed hardly to have been disturbed. That steel fence post had driven the testicle up in the scrotum, through the inguinal canal and up to nearly the top of the abdominal cavity, and the actual damage to organs and tissues had been insignificant! The closure of this second incision was done exactly like the repair of an inguinal hernia, and was completed without difficulty.

The last step needed to complete this surgery was closure of the scrotal wound. After assuring myself that the testicle was properly positioned in the scrotal sac, I closed this wound carefully, in layers, and also with the precaution of inserting a small soft rubber drain. Eventually it turned out that neither drain was necessary. Both were removed completely within a few days.

This surgery had lasted almost three hours, and it was well after midnight before I got home to bed.

The next morning was Sunday, and I slept late, so I didn't get back to the hospital for rounds until about 11:00 a.m. When I entered the patient's room, he was sitting up in bed with a wide grin on his face. He greeted me immediately with,

"Hi Doc! Boy, am I lucky. I'll be getting compensation from two places now."

"Yeah," I thought to myself, "you have no idea of just how lucky you are."

That was the moment when I nicknamed him Mr. Lucky.

After the postoperative care was completed, and I gave him his final discharge, I did not see much more of him or his family. I think perhaps that they moved from the neighborhood.

Those Damn Cows!!!!!!

The Veterans of Foreign Wars National Home is located east of town about three miles out. Originally a home for orphaned children of military veterans, its mission had been expanded to include caring for spouses of disabled veterans and their children. To raise money the VFW conducts a poppy sale once a year, in which it offers a small artificial poppy in exchange for a charitable donation. I remember huge numbers of these poppies being made in the basement of one of the VFW buildings by women employed from the area.

When the VFW National Home was filled to capacity, it housed almost 300 children, and a number of mothers. To help support so many people it operated large common vegetable gardens, and also operated a farm, which raised more of their food. At the southern end of its property there was a large farmstead with barns, a barnyard and livestock pens, where, among other things, they raised cattle. This emergency case is about a man who was injured one Sunday afternoon when some cows broke loose from the farmstead, and got out onto the VFW Road.

Visibility along this stretch of road was excellent. The road left the Grand River about half a mile from the VFW campus. Then it continued straight for another half mile along the front of the campus before it reached the VFW Farmstead. The full stretch of road was visible to anyone driving on it.

The accident victim was brought in to the emergency room by ambulance. He had been driving alone, and had run into two of the VFW cows at a high speed. His brand new Oldsmobile 442 sports car was badly damaged and he had killed at least one of the cows. He had suffered head injuries, and the ambulance attendants thought that he had been unconscious for a short time. I soon recognized who he was because he had a reputation, locally, for being wild and impulsive, and of having been in trouble with authorities from time to time as he went through high school. Recently, however, he held a well paying job at the Oldsmobile factory in Lansing, and with his employee discount was able to purchase the new car.

When I first examined him, he seemed dazed and not completely coherent. He had a bruise on his head and numerous lacerations of the scalp and face. I surmised that on impact his head had struck the windshield, and it was entirely possible that the blow could have rendered him temporarily unconscious. I also suspected that there was alcohol involved, but it was Sunday, and I could not smell any alcoholic beverage on his breath. I did a quick neurological review and testing, and was unable to detect any signs of brain damage, and I repeated the tests several times with the same result. There were major lacerations on his head and face, which needed to be repaired to minimize scarring and deformity, so we wheeled him into one of the operating cubicles in the emergency room so that I could properly repair them.

The repairs were done under local anesthesia, by injecting the anesthetic agent where it was needed. I explained that he would feel the initial needle prick at each repair site, and that if he felt anything more he should tell me immediately. The patient seemed rational and cooperative, and as time continued to pass I became more and more confident that he had sustained no significant brain damage. The repairs, carefully done to promote healing with a good cosmetic effect, took almost two hours, during which time I frequently asked questions of the patient, mainly to make certain that he had not lost consciousness, and to be sure that he remained mentally alert. I had almost finished when the patient suddenly volunteered the information.

"I saw those damn cows from a long way off! I tooted my horn! I tooted and tooted and tooted and tooted, but those damn cows just didn't get out of the way!!!"

Shell Fragments???

One Sunday afternoon in the late spring, as I was preparing to leave the emergency room after caring for several minor cases, four men in their late twenties arrived in big hurry and a somewhat agitated state.

The one in the lead came walking up to me holding up his left arm. His hand was gone, and protruding from the circle of ligaments that normally hold the wrist together were all of the tendons from the forearm muscles that run into the hand to produce its many complex movements. There are a lot of them, and the gross appearance was similar to a bouquet of wilted flowers in which the stems drooped over the edge of the vase in all directions. There was very little bleeding and the man showed no signs of shock.

The second man came in limping with obvious lacerations of his left thigh, but also showed no sign of severe blood loss or impending shock.

The other two denied being severely injured.

These men were visiting from somewhere in the Detroit area. They said that they were using dynamite to blow some tree stumps out of an old orchard by the nearby Grand River, and as they were all standing in a circle at the river's edge, a stick of dynamite exploded while the first man was holding it in his hand. It crossed my mind that they were possibly dynamiting fish, which is strictly illegal. They came to the hospital immediately in their car.

I examined all of them quickly. The man with the multiple lacerations of his thigh had wounds that resembled war wounds made by hand grenades. I had an x-ray made, and there, deep in the anterior muscle mass of the thigh were two things that should not have been there. They were large pieces of bone from the hand of the man who had held the dynamite when it exploded.

The injuries of the other two men were so minor that formal medical treatment was not needed, so I was actually faced with only two real and urgent problems. The foreign bones should be removed from the man's thigh as soon as possible to avoid infection and later complications, and the man, who had blown his hand away, needed surgical treatment soon to prepare a good stump for a working prosthesis. I discussed this with him, and pointed out that his treatment would require multiple visits to medical facilities before it was finished, and it would therefore be best to be cared for close to where he lived. The man agreed, and after a few phone calls, he was on his way to the University Hospital in Ann Arbor, Michigan.

We treated the other man in our hospital right away. Our surgical team arrived quickly, and under general anesthesia I explored the wounds in this patient's thigh. The foreign bone fragments were large, sharp-edged pieces, each of which comprised the bulk of a metacarpal bone, and the wounds that they caused were much like the shell fragment wounds I had seen on the battlefield in World War II. Fortunately the actual damage to muscle tissue was minimal, and the bone fragments were easily removed. I kept this patient in the hospital for a few days, and was quite satisfied that he was healing well when I discharged him to his doctor in the Detroit area with a written summary of everything we had done for him.

Quick Draw?

This patient was a tall, thin man, about thirty years old, whose problem arose suddenly on another Sunday afternoon. He did not live in our hospital area but was visiting his girl friend, who did live nearby. He arrived at the hospital emergency room in some physical pain and much mental anguish, because he thought that he had shot "it" off. He owned a long-barreled 22 Cal. Pistol, and was showing it off to his girl friend when the accident occurred. He had slid the barrel down under his belt, inside his trousers, and was trying to show her how fast he could "draw" and be ready to shoot, when the gun fired. He suffered immediate pain in his penis and anterior left thigh, and saw blood, but was afraid to look any further.

Upon examining him I found that he had a linear wound in his thigh, which was not much more than skin deep, and a substantial wound in about the middle of his penis. The wound had gone through the top of the urethra (the tube through which the urine comes out of the body), and through the corpora cavernosa, which are a pair of tissue sacs, about the shape of a hot dog split lengthwise, which contain the mass of blood vessels which become engorged when an erection occurs.

My immediate concern was to be sure that the patient's urine had free access to the outside, because urine excreted into body tissues can cause serious trouble. Fortunately I was able to pass a fairly large Foley catheter (a tube with a balloon at its end) through the distal urethra, across the gap in the urethra, and into the bladder. With the balloon blown up inside the bladder it is difficult to accidentally pull such a catheter out.

This seemed to me to be a case for referral to an urologist, since I had never before repaired the inside workings of a penis, so I asked the nurse to phone and arrange for a transfer to one. In the meantime I would clean up and close the skin wound in the thigh under local anesthesia.

When I finished the nurse reported that she had been unable to locate an urologist, so I personally got busy on the phone, and learned that most of the local urologists had gone to a urology meeting in California. If any were left in the area they were not available to the phone.

What to do?

I decided that I would have to repair this penis myself, so I called Dr. Sherman for the anesthesia, and mobilized the surgical team.

Actually the repair was not very difficult. I used the finest chromic catgut suture material that was available. I recognized the inner surface of the urethra (the mucosa) and carefully closed it over the catheter. The strength and thickness of the outer surface of the corpora cavernosa came as a pleasant surprise, and I found it easy to close and to accurately stitch the torn edges together. Then came the loose superficial issue, and finally the skin.

Post-operatively the Foley catheter stayed in place for a whole week, and after I removed it the patient was soon able to urinate normally. There was a bit of a problem in preventing erections, which I feared would tear out stitches and disrupt the wound closure.

In due time I discharged him to his home, which was somewhere south of Jackson Michigan, with dire warnings to treat "it" gently for six more weeks, so that the tissues would have enough time to heal solidly. I asked him to let me know if he should have any trouble, and in any case to stop in when he visited our area to let me know how he was getting along.

He did appear in my office some four or five months later, and greeted me with a great big grin.

"How has "it" been?" I asked.

"Just fine," he replied. "The only thing that's different is when I get an erection "it" is crooked, and my girl friend just loves it!!!!!"

Is he dead yet?

At about eight o'clock one evening during the winter on Highway M50 & M99 not far from the hospital a very violent collision occurred between two cars. One carried three inebriated men, who were brought by ambulance into the emergency room, one by one. All had been somewhat bruised and shaken up, but after examining each one carefully I could find no evidence of serious injury. All three were able to stand up and walk.

The driver of the car seemed to be the most inebriated of the three. His speech was most slurred. He staggered the most. He was cooperative, but his answers to my questions didn't always make sense, and I worried that he might have a closed head injury, so I decided to obtain a blood alcohol level right away. Because this service was not available in our small hospital, I made arrangements to have it done on an emergency basis at the Sparrow Hospital Laboratory, and sent the blood sample over by one of the hospital employees acting as courier. I requested that as soon as the result was ready, I wanted to be called.

In the other car involved in the accident the driver was not severely hurt. He came into the emergency room in the same ambulance as his front-seat passenger, who had the most serious injuries of all. He was a 15-year-old high school honor student who was going to school with a friend to meet his brother for an extracurricular activity in which both were participating. I recognized him immediately to be the son of special friends of mine. Because the three drunks were brought one at a time, he was the fourth to arrive, and by the time I began to examine him, his brother at the high school had heard about the accident and was already in the emergency room to support his brother. He was conscious and in great pain, most of it in his left thigh and hip. I examined him quickly, and determined that although he seemed to be seriously injured, there was nothing present which would likely be fatal. So off to X-ray he went, and the films showed a severe, comminuted (in several pieces) fracture of the femur (the big thigh bone).

It appeared to me that the best treatment for this fracture would be some type of internal fixation to hold the fragments in place while healing took place, so I turned the case over to a Lansing Orthopedic surgeon, and sent him, by ambulance, to be admitted to Sparrow Hospital.

Sadly, during his preoperative work-up there, he was found to have a chronic ear infection with pseudomonas, a bacterial infection, which was difficult to cure, and which would be almost impossible to clear up, should it get into the bone at the fracture site. So he stayed in the hospital in traction for weeks, and after the traction required another long period of leg support, and rehabilitation.

These two young men, the patient and his brother, both continued their educations to become doctors, one an obstetrician and gynecologist, and the other an emergency specialist, who has been called upon by our government to advise on the recent terrorist threats. Both of them, and their parents have told me that they decided to become doctors as the result of their experiences with me in the emergency room that evening.

Just after I had sent the ambulance on to Sparrow hospital, I received a call from the technician in the laboratory at Sparrow. The first thing he said to me was,

"Is he dead yet?"

"No," I said, "He's sitting up in a chair in the hall, and actually seems to be sobering up a bit."

"Well, his blood alcohol level is 0.4. I've never seen one that high in anyone who was still alive." (Note: A level of 0.1 is considered being "legally drunk.")

I thanked the technician, and went back into the hall to have another look at the patient. He still acted drunk, but was cooperative. I did another quick neurological examination, and examined his eye grounds carefully to be sure that there was no evidence of brain swelling. Finally I let him go off to jail, and the last view I had of him was walking away from me between two policemen toward a squad car. He still staggered a bit, but not very much.

CHAPTER XXIII

HOSPITAL INPATIENT STORIES

Actually there wasn't much humor connected with my treatment of hospital inpatients. In this chapter I have placed the few special inpatient incidents that I recall that I think are worth remembering.

The Tub Bath

In Stimson Hospital, in order to minimize the possibility of infection, it was routine, when time allowed, to require each mother-to-be to take a bath before entering the labor room. Many maternity patients bathed at home before coming in, and those who could be depended upon to be reasonably clean were excused from this requirement. The policy was actually aimed at the unwashed, of which, I am sorry to say, there were more than a few.

One day one of my obstetrical patients arrived in early labor. Bernice took her into the hospital's big bathroom, which was located not far from the nurses' station, to have her take a bath before being admitted to the labor room. Both of them were in there for a long time, and when Bernice finally came out she was laughing. She said that she had a hard time getting the patient to take the bath. After she had run about three inches of warm water into the tub, she told the patient to get in.

"I can't go in there," the woman cried, "I'll drown!"

Liquid Appendectomy

During the very early years of my practice, a woman in her early twenties came to my office with nausea, some vomiting, and abdominal pain. I examined her and found the pain to be located mostly in the lower right side of the abdomen. There was also marked tenderness to pressure in the same area, and a phenomenon which physicians call rebound tenderness, which usually indicates that there is acute inflammation of the peritoneum. These findings are typical in acute appendicitis, and to support the diagnosis I did a white blood count and a blood smear to see what kind of white blood cells were present. The count was high, and most of the white cells on the smear were polymorphonuclear leukocytes (polys). The diagnosis and the required treatment were clear. She had acute appendicitis and needed an appendectomy immediately.

Now there was a problem. Because she belonged to a welfare family, the county welfare office would not let me admit her to our Stimson Hospital. The County Hospital was Hayes-Green-Beach Hospital in Charlotte, and she would have to be admitted there. So I made the request to Hayes-Green-Beach that she be admitted there, and, I expected to be notified when she was admitted. I had long since been accepted there as a staff member, and I planned to operate there as soon after her admission as possible.

By dinnertime that evening I had not yet heard anything from Hayes-Green-Beach, so I called there to ask about my patient. She had not arrived, and the hospital had not received clearance from the County Welfare Department to admit her. So I tried to find the patient.

The family was poor and no phone was listed for them. When I called the phone number she had given for my records at the office, I was notified that the phone was "out of service." I worried about her during the night, and was somewhat relieved when she returned to my office in the middle of the next morning. She was still very ill, had pain as before, and now had a significant fever. When I examined her abdomen again, there was still much tenderness in her right lower quadrant, and now I thought I could feel a tender mass there. It was even more urgent that something more be done to get her into a hospital, but now I was thinking that the treatment must be "drainage of an appendiceal abscess", followed by an appendectomy perhaps three or four months later. She had been told to wait for the hospital to call her, and she had received no call.

In desperation I decided to approach the Welfare Department from a political angle. The supervisor for the township in which my patient lived was an elderly gentleman named Hugh Hall, who lived in the northern part of Eaton Rapids. I had had some previous contacts with him, and he had always treated me well. Late that morning I stopped at his home, where he also had a small home office, and explained the situation to him.

When he heard my patient's family name, he bristled.

"If we took the hides of that whole family, and spread them out on the wall, and sold them all at a dollar per square inch, they would still owe the County money!"

Our conversation continued, and I explained the circumstances of my patient's illness. By late that afternoon she had been admitted to Hayes-Green-Beach, and I had been notified sometime near the end of my afternoon office hours. That evening I skipped supper, and drove to Charlotte to see her, wondering just how sick she would be when I got there.

When I entered her hospital room I noticed immediately that she looked better. Her fever had subsided to a low-grade level, and she reported that most of her severe pain was gone. Shortly after she had arrived in her hospital room, the pain suddenly lessened. When I examined her abdomen I found that the mass I had felt before was still there and was still very tender, but it was definitely smaller. Some rebound tenderness remained, but it also seemed to have decreased.

At first I was amazed at the sudden change in the patient's condition, and couldn't explain it. Then after putting the pieces of the story together again, it dawned upon me that this sequence of events was very similar to what had happened whenever I had lanced a large boil or drained the pus from an abscess. The sudden relief of pain and prompt reduction of fever were typical. I thought back on a case that one of my colleagues had had, of a woman with a severe low pelvic abscess. Dr. Wadley had been consulted, and he operated immediately, to punch a hole from within the rectum into the abscess cavity to drain the pus. This patient's response was a quick relief of pain, a rapid reduction of fever, and copious evacuation of almost pure pus through the rectum, and in time this woman returned to reasonably good health.

It seemed clear to me that my patient had ruptured her appendiceal abscess, but where did the trapped pus go? Scattered into the abdominal cavity, it would cause severe widespread peritonitis, which would probably be fatal. It was certainly possible that this had happened when the pain had suddenly lessened, and that this might be "the calm before the storm." She could have a "belly full of pus and bacteria", in which case she would become very much sicker in a few hours. It also occurred to me that the abscess may have possibly eroded and ruptured through bowel wall into the caecum, and the pus was draining that way. If true, the pus could finally make its exit from the body through the colon with the feces.

In any case, this was not the time to attempt an appendectomy, which would involve distorted anatomy, be difficult to do, and would certainly stir things up and probably spread infection in the patient's abdomen. With pressure within the abscess cavity relieved, however, there was a good chance that the drainage established was good enough to allow the infection to clear. Operating now would make the patient sicker, and all kinds of bad things could happen.

So I cancelled the surgery and put the patient on an antibiotic schedule, which was very powerful for those times. She received a combination of penecillin and streptomycin by injection, and full doses of tetracycline (Terramycin) by mouth. I saw her in the hospital every day, and every day she looked and felt better. After her discharge from the hospital I followed her progress closely for several weeks, until I felt that she was out of danger.

Through the years after this illness I saw the patient in my office from time to time, and never did any problem arise in her abdomen. Then, many years after the incident, I had the opportunity to operate upon her again to identify the nature of an ovarian mass. By this time the patient was menopausal, and her children were grown. Also she was no longer a welfare patient.

At this second operation there was no sign of malignancy about which I had worried beforehand. When I examined the caecum (the part of the large bowel where the appendix is attached) and its surrounding tissues in some detail, there were a few old adhesions present, but fewer than I had expected. I followed the stria (stripe), which runs down the front side of the caecum to the base of the appendix, and found that it disappeared into an area of firm scar tissue on the bowel wall. There was no appendix there, but below this scar I found the remaining tip of the appendix. It was less than one inch long, and was hanging on a small slip of mesoappendix containing one very small artery, which was keeping it alive. I removed this small bit of useless tissue, lest it cause trouble in the future.

Throughout the years before this second surgery I occasionally discussed this case with my colleagues, especially when we were facing a case with similar conditions. We jokingly referred to the patient as the girl who had had a "liquid appendectomy". Now, after a good many years had passed, and I had done a second operation, I could assure her that she had indeed had a "liquid appendectomy", and that most of what had once been appendix had passed out of her body in the fecal stream.

Acute Myocardial Infarction

Whenever people report that someone of their acquaintance had a "heart attack" they are usually speaking about **acute myocardial infarction**, which is really a "stroke" suffered by the heart. When one of the arteries in the heart suddenly becomes occluded, the heart muscle fibers that were being fed by it die, and the function of contraction and relaxation that they had, dies with them.

In a common "stroke" an artery in the brain becomes occluded or ruptures, and the nerve cells being fed by it die. The nerve cells are no longer able to send out the electrical signals, which command muscle contraction and relaxation, and the muscle fibers that they control become totally paralyzed. Depending upon the amount of the resulting muscle paralysis, the patient's ability to move becomes impaired.

When an artery in the heart becomes occluded, the heart muscle fibers that were being fed by it die and lose their ability to contract. The function of the heart becomes instantly impaired. Depending upon how much of the heart muscle is dead and in what area of the heart it is located, various "conditions" or heart diseases are the result. When a relatively large part of the total heart muscle dies from an occlusion, the heart is no longer able to adequately pump blood through the blood vessels of the body, and the individual's demise usually follows quickly.

The ordinary symptoms of acute myocardial infarction are easily recognized. Most commonly it begins with severe chest pain directly under the breastbone, which quickly extends upward into the shoulder and down the left arm. Usually there is noticeable sweating. Whatever signs and symptoms follow depends upon the size and severity of the infarct (the dead area in the heart wall). Although today these symptoms are normally recognized for what they herald, they were not generally recognized until the 1930s. Before then patients were commonly diagnosed as having "acute indigestion," and this diagnosis is often found as the cause of death on early death certificates. Now we know that it should probably have been myocardial infarction.

The body cannot replace the heart muscle that dies from infarction with new heart muscle, but if the patient as a whole survives, the dead heart cells are reabsorbed and replaced with connective tissue cells, which ultimately turn into scar tissue that remains in place permanently. In myocardial infarction it is this "healing" period, when what was once living, active heart muscle is being absorbed and replaced with scar tissue, that is critical, and what happens during this time often determines whether the patient lives or dies. The heart cannot stop beating during this process in order to rest and heal, but must continue pumping blood, in sufficient volume and with sufficient force and speed, to sustain the patient's life. Fortunately the heart can continue to function adequately with a portion of its muscle dead and not working, but during a critical period in the process of the healing and replacement of the dead muscle, many kinds of complications can occur which can result in the patient's demise.

Serious results of acute myocardial infarction include early death because there is not enough live heart muscle remaining to sustain the blood circulation. Early death also occurs when the dead area of the heart wall includes some of the critical electric paths needed to operate to control the heart rate and rhythm. This may lead to ventricular fibrillation in which individual muscle fibers and small portions of heart wall contract at random with no coordination with each other. The net effect is about the same as a total paralysis of the heart muscle, and results in the inability of the heart, even an otherwise only mildly damaged heart, to sustain the rhythmic beats needed for life sustaining circulation. Rupture of the heart through the dead wall tissues may also occur, and means almost instant death. Late death from congestive heart failure occurs when the remaining active heart muscle is no longer strong enough to pump the minimum amount of blood necessary to sustain life.

In the days when our Eaton Rapids Community Hospital was new I admitted an elderly man through the emergency room with the typical history of an acute myocardial infarction. It was the first time I had seen him as a patient. His EKG (electrocardiogram) tracing had an ominous appearance, and I suspected that a large portion of his heart muscle had died. An admission chest x-ray confirmed my impression from my physical examination that his heart was grossly enlarged. Actually it was so big that the size of it surprised me.

In those days treatment consisted of strict bed rest and total avoidance of exertion or excitement, so that theoretically the heart would be called upon for only the minimum amount of work needed to sustain life. The administration of oxygen and the relief of pain with morphine or other narcotics were also considered crucial in the treatment. At that time it was believed by most doctors that oxygen administered in high concentrations in an oxygen tent was the best way to get the highest concentration of oxygen into the patient.

Normally this treatment would be carried out for a number of days before the patient would be allowed any physical activity. First he would be allowed to feed himself. Then in another day or two he would be allowed to get up into a chair, and if that were well tolerated, he would be allowed up to the toilet at will. As long as there were no setbacks or symptom recurrences, physical activity was gradually increased, but it was often two or three months before the patient was allowed to exercise up to the level that his damaged heart could tolerate.

This is the way treatment of my patient was begun. Because he had a very large heart I surmised that he had had some type of heart problem before he suffered this infarct. I was particularly afraid that he would go into heart failure, so I started to give him digitalis on a schedule designed to slowly raise its level in the blood to final treatment levels over a relatively long period of time. The patient seemed to respond well, but still, I was uneasy about him.

Since admission my patient had been constantly at strict bed rest in the oxygen tent with a high flow of oxygen going into it. During his third night in the hospital at about 1:00 a.m. the nurse in charge answered a ring at the hospital emergency entrance, opened the door, and standing there was my patient wearing nothing but a flimsy hospital gown wide open in the back. The outside temperature was near zero, and a strong wind was blowing. He had become confused, left the oxygen tent, got out of bed and walked down the hall to the exit at the end of it. He then went out the door, and walked barefoot around the hospital building to the parking lot, where he found his pick-up truck. He got in intending to drive home, but when, in that winter weather, his bare bottom hit the vinyl plastic truck seat, the cold shock woke him, and he walked around to the emergency entrance to call for help.

I was called immediately and came to the hospital right away to see him. When I arrived he was back in his bed in the oxygen tent, and was most apologetic, saying that he thought he had walked in his sleep. He had no complaints except that he was cold. His vital signs and blood pressure were unchanged. I could find no reason to change his medical treatment, so I didn't. The next day on rounds he was still stable and uncomplaining, and I was able to eventually discharge him from the hospital at about the usual time for cases like his. Because of his large heart I warned him about the possibility that he might develop heart failure, and cautioned him against excessive, unusual exertion.

After this hospitalization I followed the patient in my office for at least another ten years. He always had the unusually large heart, but remained active and cared for himself until he moved away from our area. It is sometimes amazing to me how well a body can get along with what seems to be a major physical impairment.

Refrigeration Anesthesia

Early in my practice the doctors were continually looking for new things that would make treatment easier for us and/or for the patient. We saw it as a big risk if it became necessary to anesthetize one of our patients with serious illness, because general anesthesia was not well tolerated by such people, and we were ever fearful that it might cause or lead to someone's death. Some of the practices we adopted successfully also were of great practical use for other patients, and, once mastered, we did not hesitate to use them on other patients, whenever the need arose.

A good example of such an innovation was the injection of local anesthetic such as Novocaine into a fracture site, a procedure which no one did in my early days out of fear of contaminating a fracture site and causing a very difficult to cure bone infection. It was easy to do. After the skin was thoroughly sterilized, the needle on a syringe full of anesthetic solution would be pushed through it, and advanced while injecting small amounts if it until the tip went into the fracture site. Fresh fractures always bleed inside, and a gush of blood into the syringe was a positive sign that the needle tip was where it should be. The contents of the syringe were quickly injected. The anesthetic agent was quickly disbursed through the blood pool at the fracture site, and in less than a minute the pain would be gone.

This allowed enough time to painlessly reduce the fracture, check the fragment positions by x-ray, and reduce it again, several times if necessary, until the best reduction possible could be achieved. Opposed to undergoing a general ether anesthetic, this was a godsend for older patients whose health was a bit precarious.

Often we would be faced with a necessity or a desirability to do major surgery for elderly patients in very poor health. In the early days of my practice, because these patients did not tolerate general inhalation anesthesia well, we tried to avoid surgery altogether, because we suspected that quite a few of them would die from the complications caused by the anesthesia. While I was still a student in medical school at the University of Michigan I had seen a mid-thigh leg amputation done on a very old diabetic man who was considered to be a very bad risk for tolerating any anesthetic. The amputation was done under refrigeration anesthesia, and it was quite a revelation to me. While the patient was propped up on the operating table with completely stable vital signs, and while he chatted with the anesthetist the whole time, the surgeons painlessly removed his refrigerated leg without any indication that the rest of his body had reacted in any way.

The first patient in this story was a thin, wiry man in his eighties, who had advanced arteriosclerosis, and had such poor circulation in his legs that he was showing early signs of gangrene in one of his feet. He was not diabetic, but did have significant arteriosclerotic heart disease, to the degree that we worried that a heart attack or heart failure might be imminent. Treatment was begun with vasodilating drugs, therepeutic doses of vitamins, and hours of elevation of the limb. There was no improvement. In a few weeks an ulcer developed on his foot, and the foot became very painful. Multiple pain medications were needed, including narcotics, and even these did not seem to be able to control the pain without robbing the patient of a portion of his senses. I suggested amputation to get rid of the pain. He didn't want that, in spite of the fact that I thought he could be fitted with an artificial leg and would be able to walk painlessly again.

As time passed, everything we tried for treatment did not seem to bring about any improvement. The forefoot turned black, and some swelling was going up above the ankle into the leg. The pain was increasing, and narcotics could not relieve it all. Finally the patient had had enough and agreed to amputation.

This immediately brought up the question of what kind of anesthetic to use. None of us were enthusiastic about giving any kind of a general or spinal anesthetic to this old man, who we thought was likely to die if he experienced even a moderate period of surgical shock.

The leg amputation in Ann Arbor under refrigeration anesthesia came to mind. I looked up all of the information available about refrigeration anesthesia in the library, including a detailed description of the procedure itself that I found in a relatively recent textbook. I thought that it would be ideal for this patient. I explained the procedure to the patient and his family, and said I would like to try it for him. He agreed to it, and I hurried about gathering equipment and researching the technique once more in the library.

Because the tissues below the knee were so close to death that if they were cut, they probably would not heal, and would make necessary a second and perhaps a third operation before the treatment was finished. I explained to the patient and his family that, in order to try to avoid such a problem, we should do an above the knee amputation. Again he agreed, and was soon admitted to our hospital.

On the morning of the surgery I got up at 4:00 a.m., and went immediately to the hospital. The patient had already received the preoperative narcotic injection I had ordered the night before. It was wintertime and cold outside, and there was a large supply of crushed ice on the back loading dock of the hospital. First we used a large rubber sheet to make a bag-like structure to hold the ice around the leg. I placed a tight tourniquet just above mid thigh to occlude the circulation in the leg. We poured crushed ice on to the rubber sheet, and put the patient's leg on it. Then we lifted up the edges of the sheet, filled the whole with more crushed ice, and wrapped the leg up in the large mass of crushed ice. I slipped a long laboratory thermometer in next to the patient's skin below the tourniquet, and was glad to see that it soon registered the temperature right where it should be.

The amputation was scheduled for 8:00 a.m. so the patient's leg would be immersed in the ice 2 ½ to 3 hours. We would theoretically have about 45 minutes to complete the operation. Actually this patient's leg was so small and thin that I was sure I would not need the whole time for the surgery, and I was also sure that the leg had been cold enough, long enough to be ready for surgery for at least an hour before we took him in to surgery.

We wheeled the bed into the operating room, took the patient out of the ice pack and placed him on the operating table, where we prepared the skin of the thigh with antiseptic solutions and alcohol, and put the leg into a heavy sterile bag before we placed it down on a sterile sheet on the operating table. Then we applied the sterile drapes that we normally use for most surgeries to protect the operative site from contamination. The surgical instruments were kept in sterile ice water, to keep the surgical site as cold as possible as long as possible. I started immediately. An anterior skin flap was made and peeled upward enough to expose the muscle mass. The muscle mass was cut across quickly just a bit higher than the level at which the skin had been cut. The same thing was done on the backside of the leg, and now the big bone of the thigh was exposed. With a tool called a periosteal elevator I peeled the membrane of the bone upward, and then used the bone saw to cut the bone in two and remove the leg from the operative field. Then I used a bone rasp (a file) to smooth the edges of the bone left behind, and put sterile "bone wax," a paraffin-like substance, into the marrow cavity to seal its contents inside. There was no bleeding during any of this because the tourniquet was still in place. Next I found the big arteries and veins in the front half and in the back half of the leg and tied them off to control the main bleeding when the tourniquet was removed. Likewise I tied off the big nerves that had been cut to try to prevent what we called amputation neuroma, and perhaps keep the patient from later on feeling phantom pain in the foot that isn't there. Then with quickly placed catgut stitches I sewed the amputated ends of the front muscles to those of the back muscles, and finished by closing the rest of the tissue layers over a small rubber drain and finally closed the skin. The patient was awake through the whole procedure and had no pain or aberrations in pulse or blood pressure. We put a pressure dressing on the stump held in place with a large elastic bandage, and moved him back into his bed, with a thermometer tucked into the edge of the bandage and a ring of ice bags surrounding it. The ice bags alleviated much of the postoperative pain and were removed gradually over several days.

Postoperatively this patient did very well. He lived for about two years before gangrene began in his other foot, and this time he asked to have it amputated. At the time our small medical group was literally swamped with work, so the patient agreed to go to the University of Michigan Hospital to have this second leg amputated. He went, had the surgery and was home again in good time, now minus both legs. He was so small and thin that in this state I estimate that he weighed only about 75 lbs, and, with his skinny arms on the arm rests of his wheel chair, he could hoist himself in and out of bed, on and off the toilet, and do many other things that seemed to still make his life worthwhile.

The second patient in this story was an obese, severely diabetic woman in her sixties who was admitted to our hospital by Dr. Cyril Hanft, of Springport, Michigan. She had extensive gangrene of both feet, which was probably not as painful as it might have been, because she was diabetic and the nerves in the lower limbs were impaired by diabetic neuropathy, a common affliction of people with advanced diabetes. Dr. Hanft asked me to see her to see if I might agree to use refrigeration anesthesia to amputate both legs. We discussed the case between us, and decided to try it. We would pack both legs in ice at the same time, and operate on both at the same time with me doing one leg, and Dr. Hanft doing the other by following my lead as I did it on my side of the table.

We explained the plan to the patient and her family, and they agreed to have both legs done this way.

Because this lady's legs were over twice the size of my previous patient's leg, I decided to allow a little more time for the legs to cool down, so that morning I got up even earlier than before. The procedure was carried out just as it had been done on the previous case, only this time we iced both legs. This time we had two extra nurses scrubbed in, and did both legs in a single, large sterile operating field. The patient was placed on the operating table. The skin preparation and application of sterile drapes was quickly accomplished. I started on the left leg, and Dr. Hanft carried out exactly the same steps at the same time as I did them on the right leg. The procedures were done in exactly the same way as I had done them on my previous patient. All went well, and both amputations were accomplished quickly, before the patient felt any pain. The stumps were dressed and elastic bandages applied. The patient was transferred to her hospital bed and both stumps were ringed with multiple ice bags. The patient remained awake throughout the operation, and there were no aberrations of pulse or blood pressure. We were quite satisfied with what we had done.

For the next several days I saw this patient several times a day. Her progress was remarkably good. Postoperative pain, partially controlled by the ice bags, responded well to narcotics. The ice bags were gradually decreased in number and were completely removed on the 4th post-operative day. The diabetes was well controlled with diet and insulin. Due to her large size this patients arms were not strong enough to lift her own weight in and out of a chair, and I was thinking that she might have to spend the rest of her life, or until she could achieve a normal weight, in a convalescent home.

On the sixth post-operative day I received a frantic call from the nurse at the hospital. This patient had summoned the nurse, complained of a severe, crushing chest pain with radiation down the left arm, and then lost consciousness. I said to see if they could get an EKG tracing, and I would come immediately. When I arrived about five minutes later, I found the patient dead. There was no EKG pattern. I eventually signed her out as having died of acute myocardial infarction.

On my way home I thought about the case. Nature had spared an obese, legless, diabetic woman from a miserable existence, and had spared me from the fact that our treatment had been a scientific success, but probably a social blunder. I felt better.

A Strange Case of FUO

FUO is an acronym that I learned to use during my internship. It meant Fever of Unknown Origin, and it was frequently recorded in medical records when the patient had a fever for which there was no good explanation. Many FUOs cleared up by themselves and remained a mystery forever, but occasionally one would progress until whatever was causing the fever became obvious to someone.

Dr. Bert VanArk admitted such a patient into the old Stimson Hospital, and after a couple of days without an explanation for the fever, he asked me to see her.

The patient was a high school girl, and was the daughter of one of the pharmacists who owned one of the drug stores downtown. Her illness had begun two days before admission with a sore throat, a mild headache and some nausea. For her sore throat she had taken penecillin lozenges, which were apparently freely available to her, and it cleared up quickly. The headache also cleared up, but mild nausea persisted off and on, and the fevers continued, varying from 99 to over 103 degrees F. Dr. Bert had done a blood count which showed the white cell count elevated with a left shift. This normally indicates that significant infection is present somewhere in the body. A chest x-ray on admission was normal, and showed the lungs to be clear.

After questioning the girl carefully without extracting any more significant information, and carrying out a general physical examination I, too, was stumped. She still complained of recurrent bouts of mild nausea, but had not vomited. Her throat was no longer sore. Concerned that some important infection was being overlooked,------ perhaps pus under pressure somewhere, I examined her carefully. There was no evidence of ear or throat infection, and no tenderness to pressure over the sinuses. Her neck was not stiff. A quick neurological examination failed to reveal any deficits. Her heart was normal, without any murmurs. Her chest was clear. There were no tender areas or masses in her abdomen, and the bowel sounds were normal. She looked like a healthy young woman with a fever, and I also could not make any better diagnosis than FUO. I considered that she might have a pelvic infection, but doubted it because with the fever and high white count I should have found at least some tenderness in the lower abdomen, and I didn't.

As I was going over the case in my mind and trying to decide whether or not to do rectal and pelvic examinations on this teen aged girl, an idea came into my mind. This was a druggist's daughter who worked in her father's drug store, and had free access to penecillin lozenges. She had admitted taking them for about two days before her hospital admission, and when I questioned her again, she admitted that she had taken quite a few. Could she have some major infectious disease, which had been attenuated by the penecillin that she took? In those days blood cultures were not done routinely. I looked at her nail beds and skin for petechiae, and there were none. I listened to her heart again, and there were no murmurs. I checked her neck again and there was no nuchal rigidity or stiffness.

On a hunch, I decided to do a spinal tap in spite of the paucity of signs and symptoms, and there I hit pay dirt. The spinal fluid was opaque with pus cells. On a smear they were seen to be mostly polymorphonuclear leukocytes, and on the smear there were also diplococci, which turned out to be gram negative when I made a gram stain.

The diagnosis was clearly meningiococcus meningitis. Penecillin was then the drug of choice for treatment, but I wondered if the microbes had been made somewhat resistant to it by the patient's consumption of penecillin lozenges. Sulfadiazine had been the drug of choice during World War II. Since the patient was not vomiting we started her on a full course of it by mouth, and also gave her more than the usual dosage of penecillin parenterally. She made an excellent recovery and was completely well without any sign of sequelae in about three weeks.

Chiropractor Referrals

Chiropractic treatment had remained a mystery to me ever since, at the age of six or seven years, I had visited one with my father. I wasn't exactly aware of what the chiropractor was doing, or why, but even at that young age I gained the impression that there was a lot of deceit and hokum in the chiropractic treatments and the explanations given for them. I learned a bit more about it as I went through medical school, and all that I learned then served to reinforce my biased bad opinion of chiropractic. Later, in my medical practice I saw patients that had been treated by a chiropractor, and I was always curious about their complaints and the advice and treatment they had been given. There seemed to be a common thread through the chiropractic advice,----- that one treatment or "adjustment" would never be enough for a cure, and patients were advised to immediately schedule as many as a dozen visits to the chiropractor's office at so many dollars per visit.

There also seemed to be several common threads running through the chiropractic claims. That the patient's spine was "out of line" and was the cause of the many complaints was, to me, preposterous. The claims that adjusting the spine would cure these complaints, and many others, were equally preposterous. I suspected that patients were often led to believe that they had diseases that they actually did not have, and then claims were made that chiropractic treatment cured them. Worse yet, the claims that chiropractic adjustments would cure organic diseases such as chronic infections, tuberculosis, and organic heart disease, were to me outright lies. I have always wondered, and I still do wonder, whether or not the chiropractor actually believes all that he tells his patients. Much of the time I believe that he does, and at other times I can only wonder about it.

The only chiropractor that to my knowledge ever referred any patients to me was the one in Eaton Rapids. He owned one of the old mineral bath hotels, and had his office in it. He still offered mineral baths and apparently had some customers for them. One morning he called me saying that he had rented a room to an elderly woman who had once been a housemother at the Veterans of Foreign Wars National Home, which was located some three miles from town. She had become ill, and he had been treating her as best he could, but she continued to get worse. He was very worried. Would I please come right away?

When I arrived with my medical bag, we went up to the second floor into the patient's room, and there was a wondrous sight to see. There was a big four-poster bed, with four very tall posts, in the room. Clothesline had been tied to the top of each post, connecting them in a square. Large blankets were hung from the lines on all four sides, forming a large cubicle with the bed inside. Several very bright lights and several heat lamps were suspended above the cubicle, including one big one for which the chiropractor had a special name. It appeared to be some kind of an infrared lamp, with a large output of heat. I pulled one of the blankets aside immediately, and there, lying unconscious on the bed, was the patient. The smell of diabetic acidosis permeated the cubicle, so I knew immediately what the diagnosis was. I could not rouse her, so I took a rectal temperature, and found it to be something over 107 deg. F. The prognosis for survival was not good.

We removed all of the heat lamps and blankets immediately, and applied some cool wet towels to the patient's body as we waited for the ambulance. I phoned the hospital to have some ice bags, a syringe with insulin, and some intravenous fluids ready. In less than ten minutes she was in bed in the hospital with an IV containing insulin, glucose and saline running. With a catheter in the bladder we found that the urine test showed a large amount of sugar. We kept up measures to cool the body down, but in spite of all we did, the patient died about an hour after admission.

My second referral from this chiropractor happened to be his wife. When he called, he explained that she had excessive vaginal bleeding, and he was treating her with adjustments and some kind of a heat and massage machine, which he applied to her lower abdomen. He explained that he had already stopped the bleeding several times, but every half-hour or so, she would start bleeding from the vagina again.

When I arrived and saw her I was greatly alarmed. She was pale and sweaty, and had a rapid pulse. I quickly learned that she had been bleeding for several days, but that the bleeding had suddenly become worse. I examined her abdomen and could palpate a huge irregularly shaped fibroid uterus, which was most likely the cause of the bleeding. The chiropractic treatment had never stopped it. It was obvious to me that this uterus had been bleeding steadily from the beginning. When the vagina filled with blood and bleeding appeared externally, the treatments would serve to express the blood and clots from the vagina. The external appearance of blood would cease until the vagina became filled up once more. Then the cycle would be repeated.

Surgical intervention was needed quickly, and most likely blood transfusions would be needed to save her life. Because quick transfusion was beyond the capability of our small hospital, I decided upon an emergency referral, and fortunately I was able to reach the gynecological surgeon that I considered most capable in Lansing by phone. I explained the urgent circumstances to him, and told him that I thought she would need some blood replacement before surgery, but then there was no point in delaying the surgery any further. To stop the bleeding, the removal of the useless fibroid uterus would be necessary.

We sent the patient to the Lansing hospital in a hurry, with sirens wailing. She got there in good time, and her course of treatment was about as I thought it would be. The story has a happy ending. She recovered, returned home, and had many more years of good life.

Odors in Medical Practice

An odor may play an important role in the way a physician works out the correct diagnosis for a patient. Some clinicians have a good sense of smell, and seem to use it regularly. Some, who have an impaired sense of smell, don't seem to use odor in diagnosis at all, but that really doesn't matter, because there are other ways to determine what the patient has. In a previous chapter I have already noted that I was aware of the individual characteristic odors of many of the houses I entered on house calls, and that I eventually became aware of the fact that, after daughters from those houses were married and had established their own homes, the daughters' homes had characteristic odors of their own, which were very similar to those of the homes in which they had had been raised.

Most doctors recognize the foul odor of rotting flesh that accompanies gangrene, and the sweet-sour-fruity smell of the diabetic patient in a coma. Many recognize the characteristic odor of the patient with terminal uremia or liver disease. But there are other, more subtle odors associated with other disease conditions, which for the most part go unrecognized.

The smells attributed to people that we call B.O. (body odor) are not directly connected with a person's health, but rather are a reflection upon his personal hygiene. Most patients who came into my office had no discernible body odor. Others were questionable, but one had to be right up close to them in order to detect it. Then there was the occasional patient about which there was no doubt. Whenever one of them entered, everybody in the room knew it.

Through the years objectionable personal body odor seems to have gradually declined to the point where today it has almost disappeared. It was more prevalent in the days when baths were taken and underwear changed only about once a week. Indeed, now many young people like to take daily showers, wash their hair daily, and change clothing often.

The patient I shall now describe shall remain nameless in this story. He had an overwhelming B.O. and much more. Wherever he went he seemed to be engulfed in a large "cloud" of odor, some of it due to strong, but ordinary body odor, and the rest if it from the cattle barn which seemed to be his castle. Friends and neighbors had even given him a nickname, which was "Cowshit," but I believe that nobody ever used that name in his presence.

The first time I met him was on a house call. When I arrived his wife directed me to the barn where he spent most of his time. She said that he even spent many of his nights sleeping there. The barn had only a single floor, but there was a floor below it much like a walkout basement. I entered the upper floor, and noted that the entrance was at ground level on this end of the barn, but the entrance to the other end of the barn was one floor level lower, and opened into the barnyard. I found myself in a large hayloft that took up about half of the length of the barn, and was partially filled with hay. The other half of the barn was two stories high, and together with the space under the hayloft comprised the space where the cattle were kept when they were inside.

My patient was there. He was about 60 years of age, and complained about a sore that he had on his shin, which wouldn't heal. He sat down to show me, and from around his leg he unrolled a large elastic bandage. The bandage was very soiled, and under it there was a generous gob of fairly fresh cow manure. He said that he had had similar sores from time to time for about two years, but had always been able to heal them by treating them with his cow manure poultices.

The smell of the barn was pretty bad, even for me. Well-rotted compost and well rotted cow or horse manure do not smell bad. Even the odor of fresh manure isn't too bad. Some people I knew even liked it. I wondered why this barn smelled so bad, and soon learned the answer when the patient took me over to the edge of the loft to look down at the huge pile of manure below. He also showed me a chair that he had built with a large hole in its wooden seat. It looked more like a seat in an outhouse privy than a toilet seat, but there could be no mistake regarding its purpose. He had fastened it securely at the very edge of the hayloft, in such a position that when he personally used it, his "droppings" would fall directly into the center of the manure pile below.

Now I had a much better understanding of the situation. When I was in Italy during World War II, the Italian farmers used a similar system of waste disposal, and every spring would spread the mixture of human and animal manure on the farm fields. Then for about three weeks the whole countryside would have a characteristic odor similar to, but not as strong, as the one, which permeated my patient's barn.

My patient's open sore appeared to me to be an arteriosclerotic ulcer, because the pulses down in the foot were feeble. To treat it I fitted a large, soft rubber sponge to be held on the ulcer with elastic bandages in such a fashion that the soft sponge would gently massage the area as he walked. I had him come in to the office several times to follow the healing process, which took about six weeks. After that I saw him in the office occasionally with other more minor complaints.

Whenever he came to the office for anything, this patient received immediate and royal treatment, because the stench surrounding him was so strong that everyone in the building knew he was there. He usually wore dirty denim overalls, which he never took off all winter long, and his barn boots, smeared liberally with manure. There were often gobs of manure to be seen hanging out of his boot-tops. He wore long winter underwear, which he never changed. I assumed that when it wore out he discarded it, and donned new "long-johns", which he wore for a year more or less until they too, "gave up the ghost."

After a couple of years had gone by, this patient suddenly developed severe shortness of breath, was taken to the hospital and admitted. He quite obviously had congestive heart failure, and was in considerable distress when he was taken to his room to receive oxygen, so I stayed in direct attendance in case any new adverse developments occurred. A nurse and a nurse's aide were present to get him settled into the bed, and I noted that they hesitated to touch him, I believe, because he was so dirty and smelled so bad. So I started the process by removing his overalls. The women pitched in to help. The filthy "long-john" underwear had been sewed shut in the front, and had to be cut open in order to get it off. I remember being grateful that he had come in by ambulance and wasn't wearing his usual barn boots. With a little soap and water and some washrags, we cleaned him up to the point that his presence was bearable in the room, and deferred the rest of it. We put his clothing into a large bag, and I think that later someone threw it out in the trash. Our impromptu ministrations had improved his condition to the point where, after the patient had improved a little, the nursing staff could begin a more normal clean-up process

The patient responded well to treatment. After he received a diuretic, he passed quarts of clear urine. Digitalis was started and the respiratory distress cleared up in a short time. Purified digitalis preparations were then available, and I prescribed Digoxin. The patient's condition leveled out on a program, which included a daily diuretic, a definitely prescribed daily dose of Digoxin, and some diet recommendations. He was eventually discharged in good condition with his prescriptions in hand.

This story does not have a happy ending, however, because a few days later someone found old "Cowshit" in his beloved barn, stone cold, stiff, and very dead. Nearby was the empty prescription vial for one of the prescriptions I had written for him. He had obviously swallowed all of the remaining ninety-five or so pills of Digoxin at one time, and committed suicide!

CHAPTER XXIV

FOREIGN BODY STORIES

At the age of five years, shortly after I had my tonsils and adenoids removed, I made up my mind to become a doctor. In the ensuing years I paid attention to scientific and medical information whenever I came across any, and I did much reading. I had an inside track to the medical world, because my uncle, Herman A. Meinke, M.D. owned and operated a proprietary hospital in Hazel Park, Michigan, the HELENE MEINKE HOSPITAL, which he named after my grandmother. It was only about a three-mile walk from where I lived to the hospital, and after I had become about twelve years old, I was able to walk there easily, and I often did, to visit my grandmother, who lived next door, and to do odd jobs in the hospital. The chores that I did were quite menial, but I didn't mind, because I had many chances to spend time in the laboratory and to observe medicines and medical equipment.

Then when I was fourteen years old, Uncle Herman removed my appendix. Although I had been sick only about ten hours, he found that my appendix had ruptured, and he wisely placed a rubber drain into my abdomen, bringing the end of it out through the incision that he had made. The drain tube, with a large safety pin stuck through its protruding end to keep it from falling back into the abdomen, allowed the escape of pus from the abdominal cavity as soon as it formed. The tube remained in place for many days, even after I was able to return home from the hospital, and it was removed gradually by intermittently pulling about half an inch of it out, reinserting the safety pin, and trimming off the excess outer length of the protruding tube. This procedure created a wound track, which carried the pus out of my abdomen. By shortening the tube in small increments this way, the track was allowed to heal slowly, so it closed up from the inside out, without trapping any infection inside the abdomen. When the tube became so short that it literally fell out of the wound, it took only a few more days for the wound to heal up completely. This was my first lesson on foreign bodies inside the human body.

While I was still in the hospital and feeling better, I became very curious about that red rubber drain tube. The tubing looked to me like the same tubing that came with enema bags, through which enemas were given to patients. When I asked about it, one of my nurses, who had assisted with my operation, told me,

"Yes that's where the tube came from."

Uncle Herman's small hospital was located on the second floor above a row of stores on Eight Mile Road, and its operating room looked like a large, ordinary bedroom. In it were an operating table, some special lights, several instrument cabinets, some shelves containing bandages and medicines, and on a small table in one corner there was an electric hot plate.

The nurse told me that when Uncle Herman decided that a drain was needed, he had someone take the enema bag down from where it was hanging on the back of the operating room door, cut off a piece of the tubing about ten inches long, and boil it in a large pan of water on the hot plate for about ten minutes. He then placed it into the wound.

During the two or three days following my operation I became very ill, and when on the second day my fever was up a little, Uncle Herman thought I was becoming dehydrated. Probably because my abdomen was still distended, and I was still nauseated intermittently, he thought that I should have parenteral fluid, so that my gastrointestinal tract could remain at rest for a longer time.

It was the practice of the time to give parenteral fluids by a slow drip through a needle placed into muscle or subcutaneous spaces in the body. This process was called hypodermoclysis, or just clysis for short. In those days such fluids were not commercially available. Uncle Herman made his own fluids for clysis. First he distilled the water using the still in his laboratory. Then he carefully weighed chemically pure table salt (Sodium Chloride), and added it to the water in the proper amount needed to produce physiological saline solution. The solution was then sterilized in an autoclave. When administered it was run through gum rubber tubing, then through a hypodermic needle. I received the benefits of this treatment with a needle in each anterior thigh.

In those days the tubing for administering a clysis was usually cleaned, sterilized, and re-used, and the needles were also cleaned, sharpened on a whetstone if necessary, and re-used. The term, *pyrogens*, was used to describe certain trace impurities often found in fluids administered intravenously or by clysis. These fever-causing substances were believed to come from the tubing, and were very difficult to avoid or remove. Autoclaving usually was not enough to destroy them. They were even present in new tubing being used for the first time.

Obviously, I received pyrogens in my clysis. When my fever went above 104 degrees F. and I felt most miserable, my grandmother, who at the time was the hospital cook, came into the room. I remember her coming up to my bed, wide eyed, clapping her hand up to her head, and saying, in German, which was my first language,

"Quick, somebody call the photographer! This may be the last day we will see this boy alive!!"

What a way to cheer up a sick grandson!

Obviously I did not die, although full recovery took a long time. Afterward I became ever more determined to become a doctor, and it was not until I was well into my medical practice that I fully appreciated the extent of that illness that I had. The skill, knowledge, and good medical sense of my Uncle Herman had surely saved my life! Indeed, it was that piece of red rubber enema tubing that did it!

My bout with the ruptured appendix was probably the reason why I was always a firm believer in the use of drains and drainage tubes in surgery. Possibly I used them too much throughout all of my practice years. However, whenever I placed a drain into a wound when it turned out not to be actually needed, I removed it early, without causing any problems and without prolonging the patient's hospital stay.

A Surgical Tool?

The doctor, who removed my tonsils and adenoids when I was five years old, was Clarence Baker, M.D., an Eye, Ear, Nose and Throat (EENT) specialist, who treated patients in my uncle's hospital. He was also on the staffs of several large Detroit hospitals, and played golf with my father almost every Sunday morning. He told this story to my father who later told it to me.

As Dr. Baker was going in to see some patients in one of the large Detroit hospitals, he passed by the emergency room, was hailed and was asked to help the two physicians there, who were struggling with a problem. One of them was the physician on emergency call, and the other was an obstetrician, whom he had called in. The problem was a middle-aged woman with a huge white potato stuck firmly in her vagina. She couldn't get it out, became alarmed, and went to the emergency room. The doctors had unsuccessfully tried several maneuvers to remove the potato, including the use of obstetrical forceps. They asked Dr. Baker if there might be some kind of instrument that an EENT doctor might have that might help. Doctor Baker replied,

"Sit tight. I know just what you need."

He then went to the hospital kitchen and obtained the biggest corkscrew available, returned to the emergency room, and watched while the obstetrician easily removed the potato with it.

Buckshot, Glass and Other Things

During my practice years I saw a number of patients with a variety of foreign bodies embedded within their flesh. The most frequent and easiest to treat were foreign particles that were embedded into the cornea of the eye. The majority of these were caused accidentally while the patient was using a sharpening or grinding wheel. Usually these are easy to remove. After anesthetic drops have been put into the eye, they are easily dug out with an instrument called an eye spud. I often used a large bore hypodermic needle with its sharp, beveled edge to do the job. One had to be careful not to perforate the cornea, but one also had to be sure to scrape any discolored tissue out of the crater left behind, because such dirt or dead tissue could result in opaque scar forming in the cornea, which would impair vision. Otherwise the cornea of the eye usually heals rapidly and remains clear and transparent.

Other foreign body cases, which were common, included wounds caused by buckshot or BB's from an air rifle, glass, metal scraps and broken needles. Broken needles embedded in someone's flesh were a big problem, because the public occasionally read about someone running a needle into a hand and losing it, only to have it "travel" within the tissues and appear on the surface again at some distant site. Some stories even had the needle going to the heart and killing the patient. Because this was so, I removed all buried needles as soon as possible, before they had a chance to move very far. I developed a method of doing so which consisted of finding the needle under the fluoroscope, injecting local anesthetic solution to anesthetize the region, and leaving the injection needle in place with its tip against the lost needle. Then, away from the fluoroscope and out in the light again, I could cut through the skin and dissect the underlying tissues to follow the injection needle to its point, and easily find the errant needle to retrieve it. I used this same method to remove most metallic foreign bodies. These were sometimes easier to do, because, after obtaining anesthesia, I could insert the closed tip of a hemostat into the wound track and, under the fluoroscope, grasp the foreign body with it, and pull it out through the same path that it taken as it entered the flesh.

Glass particles buried in the flesh were the most difficult to remove. Most glass was invisible under the fluoroscope, although occasionally with leaded glass it could be faintly seen and fluoroscopy could be used to help in removing it. Otherwise it was necessary to do an open operation and search for it more or less blindly. It had to be successfully found before one could remove it, and this was seldom easy to do. Sometimes I elected not to remove it for fear of tearing up a lot of good, healthy tissues. In such cases the glass particle would often eventually become encysted in scar tissue and lie dormant, which is also what happens with wartime shell fragments, which are not removed from soldiers' bodies. If the glass is sharp, and not too far under the skin, it may, in time, work its way to the surface where it may be easily removed through a small nick in the skin. If the glass starts an infection in the wound, it becomes necessary to remove it to allow healing to occur, and in the presence of pus it is usually confined in the infected wound tract, and is easier to find.

Sometimes so-called foreign bodies are really not in the body at all. Examples of these include the speck of dirt or sand in the eye, the toy in the nose or ear, the stuff that people swallow that is not food, and material that may be aspirated into the lung. This type of foreign body is not actually in the body in the sense that it has invaded body tissues. It is essentially like holding a gob of mud in a closed hand. The mud in the hand, and the swallowed coin demonstrate similar situations. They may be said to be in the body, but they are not truly in the body tissues. They have not invaded any living tissue. The ones that are swallowed are not really within the body, but are within the gastrointestinal tract, which is a tube running through the body, which is connected to the outside environment at each end. It is really a portion of the outside world in which special conditions exist that make it possible for the body to gain nourishment and reject wastes. Likewise the bean in the nose and the small toy in the ear canal are not actually within the body tissues.

The seriousness of foreign body cases of this type depends upon the location and the circumstances of the foreign body. For example, before the advent of bronchoscopy, it was a death sentence for a child to aspirate a peanut into the lung. The peanut must be removed, if the child is to recover, and today this is most often done with bronchoscopy. On the other hand, all kinds of foreign bodies have been swallowed, and have in time passed on out of the rectum without harming the person. Although it always amazes me, I have seen straight pins, pieces of razor blade, broken glass, and even open safety pins pass through the gastrointestinal tract without doing any damage at all!

The Lost Penny

One day when my office was still in Stimson Hospital, a three-year-old child was brought in by his parents, who were very agitated and excited because they had seen their son swallow a penny. Upon examination the child seemed to be quite normal, so I quickly looked at him under the fluoroscope to be sure that the penny was truly in the stomach, and not in the trachea (windpipe) or esophagus (food pipe). When I saw that it was indeed in the stomach, I knew that it should pass easily in the stool. To be sure that it was safely out, I told the parents to try to recover it.

Now these parents were hesitant and seemed truly fearful that something bad would happen if they took their child home with that penny in his stomach. I soon learned why, when they told me this story:

A good friend's young child had swallowed a nickel, and was rushed to the emergency room at the Osteopathic Hospital in Lansing. He was x-rayed, and admitted to the hospital. Every three hours he was taken to the x-ray room and yet another film was taken. In this way the passage of the nickel through the intestinal tract was followed, and at about twenty-four hours, "plunk!!!" went the nickel into the bedpan.

The hospital bill was over $400.00.

My patient passed the penny at home, and the parents recovered it. My bill for the office call was $3.00.

A Swallowed Chain?

The Veterans of Foreign Wars National Home had its campus about three miles from our office, and we would occasionally see a child from there who had swallowed something unusual. Most of the items were metallic, and were easily seen on x-rays and by fluoroscope. Rarely one of the older children swallowed a collection of objects. Whatever has been swallowed and has reached the stomach will usually pass in the stools, so we usually made sure that the stuff was really in the stomach, and waited for the patient to pass it. It is remarkable that open safety pins and even straight pins seem to be passed easily without damaging the stomach or bowel.

One afternoon a fifteen year old boy from the VFW Home came to the office complaining of right lower quadrant abdominal pain, which had begun the evening before. His general and abdominal physical exams were normal, except for definite, but mild, tenderness over the region of the appendix. The white blood cell count was only slightly elevated, and the distribution of the cell varieties was about normal. He had no fever. An x-ray of his abdomen showed, in the right lower quadrant, what appeared to be a piece of a pull chain from a light socket. These chains were built of small, uniform metallic balls strung together. This piece appeared to be about three inches long and was located about where the appendix should be.

After some hours had passed and the patient's pain had become sharper, I thought I detected a hint of rebound tenderness in the painful area, which would indicate inflammation of the peritoneum. I decided to operate. The preoperative diagnosis was acute appendicitis.

At surgery I delivered the caecum and appendix into the operative field quickly and easily. The appendix did not appear inflamed, but it didn't look normal either. Its wall was swollen and puffy looking. I could feel the beads of the "chain" inside, so I completed the surgery by doing a routine appendectomy. After it had been removed we opened the appendix and found, not a chain, but about a dozen small steel balls. They were steel shot from a shotgun shell. This was the first year that the hunting laws prohibited the use of lead shot for hunting waterfowl, and required that steel shot be used instead. My patient had eaten a large meal of wild duck, and had ingested the shot with the meat. What is most remarkable to me is that all of the ingested shot was found lined up inside of the appendix. The x-ray showed none of it anywhere else in the abdomen. My patient made a good, rapid recovery

Another Case That Was Not Appendicitis

One day a middle-aged woman came to the office with a typical history and physical findings of appendicitis. There was no doubt in my mind about it, so we operated as soon as possible. Once inside the abdomen I was most surprised to find that a round cocktail toothpick, pointed at both ends had perforated the caecum (part of the large bowel) and was stuck about halfway out through the perforation. The appendix was normal, but after I closed up the hole in the bowel, I removed it, and placed a soft rubber drain into the area. The drain was necessary because she had leaked bacteria from inside of the bowel into the sterile abdominal cavity, and the drain would prevent a post-operative abscess from forming. The wound did drain pus for a time after the operation. .

Although the patient could not account for the toothpick in her bowel, she must have swallowed it. One of her hospital visitors clued me in. It seemed to be that he lady was a hard drinker who became inebriated regularly. In that condition she could have successfully swallowed that toothpick without knowing or remembering it. A week or so after the surgery we received the report from the State Laboratory that the woman's serology test was positive. I was glad that we all had worn gloves at the operation, and I concluded that, certainly, here was a lady who had washed in many waters.

Foreign Bodies in the Ears and Nose

During my practice years I saw many, many patients with foreign bodies in the ears and nose. Almost all of them were young children. Sometimes the parents seemed ignorant of the dangers imposed by these foreign bodies. In the ear crude attempts at removal could lead to a badly damaged eardrum, serious infection in the middle ear, and much loss of hearing. In the nose, snuffing a foreign body backward into the throat, posed the danger of aspirating it into the lung, which was a most serious and expensive complication. Even though some medical books recommended shoving a catheter through the nostril to shove the foreign body out through the back, I never did it that way because I was afraid of the possibility of aspiration.

There were a number of methods of removal that I liked to use, and I believe that I added a few innovations to them on my own.

Foreign bodies in the ear included, peas, beans, stones, pieces of rubber from pencil erasers, and insects, alive and dead. Live insects were an immediate emergency because the patients were seemingly going mad with the buzzing and crawling in the ear. Usually the insect was a small one, because the larger ones would crawl out by themselves very quickly. Removing them was usually easy with a small jet of water from an ear syringe, which flushed them out. The other items were more difficult. If they were small they could sometimes be flushed out, but often they were large and were wedged more or less snugly into the ear canal. To try to remove them with forceps or a hemostat would, except for the stones, cause them to break up, and if one spent enough time breaking it up one could eventually flush all of the foreign material out of the ear canal. I usually chose not to break them up, but preferred to remove them in the same way that I removed the stones.

Stones were more difficult, but I finally settled on a method that worked well for me. Sometimes I dropped a bit of local anesthetic into the ear canal. Then a drop or two of a vasoconstrictor such as neosynephrine nose drops to shrink the swollen, irritated tissues. Then using a bit of sterile lubricant I could slide a long loop of sterile tonsil snare wire along the wall of the ear canal past the stone. Once past the stone the wire loop could be opened up a bit, and the loop would then slide in behind it. By gently pulling the wire out, the loop would bring the stone out with it.

Foreign bodies in the nose were larger than those that got into the ears. Some could be removed easily with forceps or a hemostat, but where this was not possible I removed them by bringing them out forward with a tonsil snare or some similar wire loop similarly to the way I removed foreign bodies from the ear.

A Record for a Foreign Body?

I had one nasal foreign body case that was very unusual. The patient was a 63-year-old white woman who complained of pain in one side of her nose and a more than usual nasal discharge. I could see the foreign body through a nasal speculum, but I could not identify it. I extracted the history from the patient with some difficulty. She stated that she remembered clearly that when she was about three years old and growing up with her poor family somewhere in the South, she put a dried bean up her nose. She could not remember that it was ever removed. Yes she had trouble breathing through the left side of her nose, but she thought that that her nose had grown that way, and that it was normal for her.

The foreign body was greenish in color and hard. I could grasp it firmly with tweezers, and after fussing with it for a while I was able to grasp it with a small hemostat. Then with topical anesthetic and sterile lubricant, and a few instruments that I could use as tiny retractors, I was able to work it out of the nasal cavity without causing any significant damage. The specimen was circular in shape with rough edges, larger than a fifty-cent piece, but slightly smaller and thicker than a silver dollar. It was greenish-blue in color, and reminded me of a bit of copper ore I had seen in someone's collection. I could recognize nothing that looked like the original bean, but after sixty years in someone's nose, it was bound to lose its identity.

I assume that the patient recovered well. After she left my office I never saw her again.

I wonder if this might be a record for length of time for a foreign body in someone's nose?

APPENDIX A

The following article written by ***Edward B. McRee****, then President of the Ingham Medical Center in Lansing, Michigan, appeared in the spring 1984 issue of the Eaton Rapids Community Hospital newsmagazine. It was written in anticipation of Dr. Meinke's retirement from practice in the autumn of 1984, and is reproduced here with permission.*

Because He Cared...

By Edward B. McRee

President, Ingham Medical Center

Little did I know when I carefully listened to my first telephone call from Eaton Rapids, Michigan, that the voice and the place would become an integral part of the life of myself and my family. With brief introductory remarks, the man at the other end assured me that a new hospital was being built in Michigan and a position might be available in that organization if our mutual goals could be met. The caller was Albert H. Meinke, Jr., M.D.

In a few short days following that telephone call, I received in my place of work at Fort Bragg Army Hospital, three men who would become my warm friends and counselors in the ensuing years. Pilot for the airborne trio was George F. Miller, a long-time community activist and prominent businessman, and his passengers were the chairman of the hospital board and automobile dealer, L.L. McNamara and their advisor and community medical leader, Albert H. Meinke, Jr., M.D.

At the time I was struck with their zeal! The three had flown in the small private plane from Michigan to North Carolina, for the express purpose of visiting about their new hospital and the position they had available within the facility.

A few weeks later, I was to see and visit with yet more of the people in Eaton Rapids who were equally inspired and fervent about the task they had undertaken, and it was an impressive occurrence. It was on this occasion that I first met the four physicians who were to ultimately give their privately owned hospital to the new Eaton Rapids Hospital, and make a transfer of those assets to the new venture.

My introduction began in the old Stimson Hospital, and it was here that I met with Dr. Bert VanArk, the senior member of the group. With many years of medical practice behind him, he greeted me with his strong grasp and Dutch smile, as we paused to chat about the city which he was so very fond of, and to which he had dedicated most of his professional life. I soon surmised that with his dog, "Shelly" he had become a household word in the area, and that one of his favorite tasks was dispensing candy mints to the children. He cherished his daily trip to the VFW National Home where he served as mentor and friend, as well as trusted physician.

In the next office resided Doctor Bert's nephew, Dr. Herman VanArk. Suave and dapper and filled with an impish smile, the city health officer enjoyed not only popularity, but an exuberant zest for life. Always absorbed with a wide circle of friends, his style was casual and confident and he gave to the town a quality of concern and understanding that endeared him to everyone.

It had become a time of revelation for me, and as I encountered more and more people, it became increasingly evident that there was a concern for the new hospital, which was contagious.

The black and white checked tile of the lobby led to several doors, and bustling out of one, with a boyish grin and sonorous welcome, was the newest member of the group, Dr. Eber Sherman. Recently discharged from the Air Force, he located in Eaton Rapids to practice medicine with his father-in-law, Dr. Bert VanArk, and brought special talents in anesthesiology to the group, as well as his skills in the area of family medicine. His exuberance was excelled only by his drive, and I was certain that he would work diligently to forge the new and the old into a strong medical institution.

To this trio was added two other people – both of whom I would greatly respect and cherish as colleagues, the administrator of the Stimson Hospital, Bernice Bowman and the financial officer, Mary Jordan. Any recall of the formative years of the Eaton Rapids Community Hospital would be incomplete without their inclusion. It was the generousness on the part of Bernice, which made me welcome. A faithful nurse and administrator, she had for many years, capably directed the activities of the hospital and was additionally a part-owner of that institution. It was her insight which paved the way for my presence and her warmth that made my visit successful. From her I quickly discerned acceptability and support, and through my working years in Eaton Rapids I found her to be a giant of an arm upon which I leaned many, many times. It was she who paved the road so frequently for undertakings upon which I embarked, and through her winsome personality prevailed under frequently less than optimal circumstances.

Added to her kind leading was the dedication and "know-how" of Mary Jordan. A whirlwind of activity and energy, she maintained an enormous knowledge of the reimbursement system and an immense capacity for work. She too, was endowed with the ardor and fervor that characterized the thinking about the new hospital and without her help, much of what was accomplished would never have been possible.

My guide and leader through this maze of new faces and personalities was the man who initially assured me that if we could meet our mutual goals, there might be a place for me in Eaton Rapids Community Hospital. Albert Meinke. And it is because of him, that I have penned these remarks.

All that I have noted is history, nearly thirty years ago. Some of these marvelous people have passed on, others have retired. Some move within the community and continue to make distinguished contributions to the life of the inhabitants.

At this writing, our mutual friend, Albert H. Meinke, Jr. is also planning retirement. Soon he and his wife, Edmere, will release their present home, and move to their dream house on Torch Lake.

While I do not know – I strongly suspect that Doctor Meinke was the influencing voice which led to my employment. In our initial conversations, his appraisals of what was needed and what could be expected were always accurate, forever candid, and remarkably insightful. And throughout the twenty-seven years that I have known him, he has been consistent that way.

From the initial planning of how we might equip the new hospital building to this present day, when hospitals find themselves constantly examining the environment to assess their future and their livelihood – he has been an optimist. But one of his most obvious strengths has been that he was more that just an optimist – he was an educated optimist. When things seemed virtually impossible, and certainly improbable, he invariably had read something which would relate to the problem and which offered options, or the hint of an option. It was upon these pivotal points that much of the strategy for growth and expansion of Eaton Rapids Community Hospital rested and the results have been dynamic.

For every organization or group of people, there needs to be a rock, an unquenchable voice of reason and perceived guide, and he filled those shoes admirably. Ours was a small hospital in a small community – but the dynamics of achievement never evaded our doors and because he was a team player and tireless innovator, he encouraged all of us to constantly do better and try new things.

Physicians are always pressed with endless duties, but he continuously found time for those which were important to the hospital. Dozens of times he traveled to some other city or place to enlist consultants, look at new approaches, or gain insight that could benefit our institution. And while much of what was accomplished in Eaton Rapids Community Hospital was not heralded, it was still innovative and well executed. His willingness to try new things brought insightful medicine to the community.

Long before it was fashionable and/or acceptable, the practice of fathers in the delivery room was strictly routine in this community. Originating in the old Stimson Hospital, the practice preceded by fifteen years, the wave of acceptability which finally came to the majority of hospitals.

The utilization of visiting consultants to both diagnose and perform surgery in order to maintain the patients in their home community rather than being transferred to other cities, wasn't considered unusual in Eaton Rapids because it was perfunctory. It is the way of life for smaller hospitals today, as they seek to maintain their patient occupancy – but many years ago, it was only done where strong liaison occurred between physicians and great respect for the judgment of the local practitioner existed. This hospital literally grew with this practice and few appreciated that it was only because of local competency that the practice could be carried out. Albert Meinke fostered the recruitment of consulting staffs, and in so doing he brought specialists to the patient, rather than send the patient to the specialists. Always the teacher, he engendered in my thinking the understanding that one must constantly improve the knowledge base if we are to stay on the keen edge of advancement. An inveterate reader and student, he kept up with not only the trends in medicine, but the changing ways of hospitals. It was through this ardent interest that he perpetually challenged all of us to be better tomorrow than we were today.

All of his life as a practicing physician and surgeon has been memorable. In a quiet and most unobtrusive way he has given his utmost to the community. Next to medicine, his consuming public service was a long and respected tenure of the public school board. As both member and chairman, he served in this post as diligently as he practiced medicine. Again, passionate learning enabled him to make outstanding contributions and his tenacious energy greatly enhanced the role and direction of public education in this community. None of what he has done or may yet do in the future can be isolated from the help he received at home. His wife and family made immense sacrifices of time and many opportunities, when his obligations called and took precedence. Four successful and grown children attest to the capable home that Edmere managed, and to the individual strength that each possessed

Reality dictates that Eaton Rapids is losing one of its mightiest boosters and powerful assets. Others will undoubtedly fill the void and assume the mantle – but unquenchable leadership is difficult to replace and impossible to duplicate. His humor and wit will be sorely missed, and the grin a fond remembrance. The counsel and erudite composure have long been hallmarks to many people and without these qualities – many of us will be shortchanged.

But the good that he has fostered remains with the community and within the understanding and memories of many, many people. It is thus with warm wishes for joy in their new venture that we wish Al and Edmere Meinke wonderful years in the future. They have granted us more of themselves than we may deserve – but they have enriched our lives in so doing.

www.ingramcontent.com/pod-product-compliance
Ingram Content Group UK Ltd.
Pitfield, Milton Keynes, MK11 3LW, UK
UKHW051130260726
13967UKWH00010B/2963

9 781553 957454